Register Now for Online A~~ccess~~
to Your Bo~~ok~~

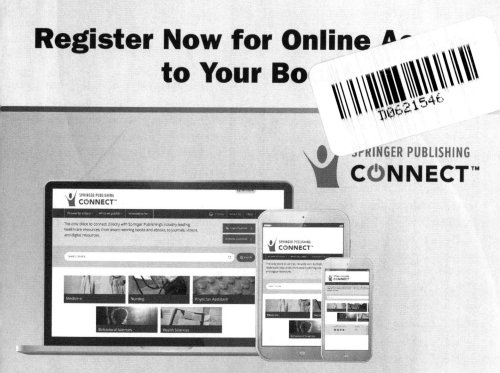

SPRINGER PUBLISHING
CONNECT™

Your print purchase of *Proposal Writing for Clinical Nursing and DNP Projects* **includes online access to the contents of your book**—increasing accessibility, portability, and searchability!

Access today at:
http://connect.springerpub.com/content/book/978-0-8261-4443-0
or scan the QR code at the right with your smartphone and enter the access code below.

7C7USJV7

Scan here for quick access.

If you are experiencing problems accessing the digital component of this product, please contact our customer service department at cs@springerpub.com

The online access with your print purchase is available at the publisher's discretion and may be removed at any time without notice.

Publisher's Note: New and used products purchased from third-party sellers are not guaranteed for quality, authenticity, or access to any included digital components.

 SPRINGER PUBLISHING
View all our products at springerpub.com

Wanda Bonnel, PhD, APRN, ANEF, is associate professor at the University of Kansas School of Nursing, Kansas City, Kansas. As a specialist in geriatrics and nursing education, she teaches courses in the master's, doctor of nursing practice (DNP), and doctoral programs, including advanced clinical residency and a project course for DNPs. She is a fellow of the National League for Nursing Academy and recipient of the Chancellor's Distinguished Teaching Award at the University of Kansas, and received the Sigma Theta Tau Regional Pinnacle Award for computer-based professional education technology. Dr. Bonnel has received multiple funded grants, including the Health Resources and Services Administration (HRSA) online Health Professions Educator Certificate program. She has published numerous peer-reviewed abstracts and articles in geriatric and educator specialty journals, including *Clinical Advisor* and *Journal of Professional Nursing*. She co-authored the textbook *Teaching Technologies in Nursing and the Health Professions* (2010). Her ongoing research interests include online learning best practices and advanced practice mentoring. Dr. Bonnel has served as grant reviewer for the National League for Nursing and HRSA and a manuscript reviewer for selected journals, and is an editorial board member of the *Journal of Gerontological Nursing*. Her recent work in the DNP advanced clinical and advanced leadership project courses provides valuable background and opportunity to identify selected student-learning needs for this text.

Katharine V. Smith, PhD, RN, CNE, is associate professor and assistant dean for program evaluation at the University of Missouri—Kansas City School of Nursing and Health Studies. Dr. Smith has received multiple grants, most of which have focused on aspects of teaching, advanced education, and nursing traineeships. Recent scholarship includes peer-reviewed publications and national presentations on the use of simulation to teach legal and ethical content. She has also co-authored the textbook *Teaching Technologies in Nursing and the Health Professions* (2010). Dr. Smith teaches in both the undergraduate and the graduate nursing programs, facilitating advanced clinical projects through the institutional review board process. She also conducts program review and site visits for both nursing and nonnursing programs and serves as a manuscript reviewer for selected journals.

Proposal Writing for Clinical Nursing and DNP Projects

Second Edition

Wanda Bonnel, PhD, APRN, ANEF

Katharine V. Smith, PhD, RN, CNE

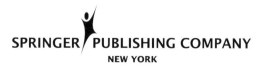

SPRINGER PUBLISHING COMPANY

NEW YORK

Springer Publishing Company, LLC
11 West 42nd Street
New York, NY 10036
www.springerpub.com

Acquisitions Editor: Joseph Morita
Compositor: diacriTech

ISBN: 978-0-8261-4442-3
e-book ISBN: 978-0-8261-4443-0

18 19 20 21 22 / 7 6 5 4 3

The author and the publisher of this Work have made every effort to use sources believed to be reliable to provide information that is accurate and compatible with the standards generally accepted at the time of publication. Because medical science is continually advancing, our knowledge base continues to expand. Therefore, as new information becomes available, changes in procedures become necessary. We recommend that the reader always consult current research and specific institutional policies before performing any clinical procedure. The author and publisher shall not be liable for any special, consequential, or exemplary damages resulting, in whole or in part, from the readers' use of, or reliance on, the information contained in this book. The publisher has no responsibility for the persistence or accuracy of URLs for external or third-party Internet websites referred to in this publication and does not guarantee that any content on such websites is, or will remain, accurate or appropriate.

Library of Congress Cataloging-in-Publication Data

Names: Bonnel, Wanda E., editor. | Smith, Katharine Vogel, editor.
Title: Proposal writing for clinical nursing and DNP projects / Wanda Bonnel,
   Katharine V. Smith.
Other titles: Proposal writing for nursing capstones and clinical projects
Description: Second edition. | New York, NY : Springer Publishing Company,
   [2018] | Preceded by: Proposal writing for nursing capstones and clinical
   projects / Wanda Bonnel, Katharine V. Smith. 2014. | Includes
   bibliographical references and index.
Identifiers: LCCN 2017017713 | ISBN 9780826144423 | ISBN 9780826144430 (e-book)
Subjects: | MESH: Clinical Nursing Research | Writing | Research Design
Classification: LCC RT71 | NLM WY 20.5 | DDC 610.73076--dc23 LC record available at https://
   lccn.loc.gov/2017017713

Printed in the United States of America by McNaughton & Gunn.

Contents

Section III: Writing Your Proposal: Adding the Detail for Proposal Completion

Appendices

Contributors for Proposal Abstracts and Project Examples

Karri Arndt, DNP, APRN
University of Kansas, Nurse Anesthesia Education, Kansas City, Kansas

Sonya Curtis, DNP, MBA, RN, CNL
Veterans Affairs North Texas Healthcare System, Dallas, Texas

Paula Israel, DNP, APRN-BC
University of Kansas School of Nursing, Kansas City, Kansas

Linda Kroeger, DNP, APRN-FNP-BC
University of Kansas School of Nursing, Kansas City, Kansas

Roberta Mansfield, DNP, FNP-BC
Washburn University School of Nursing, Topeka, Kansas

Jane Robinson, DNP, FNP-BC
Washburn University School of Nursing, Topeka, Kansas

Gwenyth Wagner, DNP, APRN-C
Health Partnership Clinic, Olathe, Kansas

Brigid Weyhofen, DNP(c) MSN, NEA-BC
University of Kansas School of Nursing, Kansas City, Kansas

Preface

As new graduate programs evolve at schools across the country, diverse student cohorts have the opportunity to enhance their skill sets in planning and writing proposals. This book shares the "must know" for gaining a set of clinical scholarship tools for writing a concise, scholarly project proposal. The purpose of the text is to provide practical guides for graduate students and advanced clinicians to organize and package their clinical projects through tight proposals.

The concept of advanced clinical projects is described broadly. All health care professionals, whether they are in direct or indirect practice roles, are, in essence, seeking to provide improved health outcomes for all populations and quality, efficient patient care. This uniqueness provides an opportunity to raise awareness of diverse important problems or concerns in various practice areas.

A well-written clinical project proposal is a form of scholarly communication and is expected in advanced practice. The text is broadly written to support diverse clinical project topics. Although the uniqueness of advanced nursing practice allows no one proposal "formula," there are guides for taking unique topics and relating these to common project models. Focus is on the use of the best evidence in projects, including synthesis of the literature for further project development.

Gaining ongoing skills for quality improvement, evaluation, and collaborative research is valued. Although clinical projects can have similarities to theses and dissertations in some cases, the clinical project proposals are much more focused on gaining best evidence for use in advancing quality patient care. Often the tools of research will be used in writing proposals, but the focus of the clinical project is to gain best use of evidence for improving clinical care. This book guides the reader in using tools gained in previous courses, such as theory, research, and statistics, to develop a sound proposal for a quality advanced clinical project. The "must know" information from these courses is reinforced, and resources for further reading are recommended.

Being a reflective clinician brings an important component to a clinical project proposal. This relates to thinking prospectively of the big picture of the project, from start to finish, so important parts are not missed. A toolkit of resources, including a project triangle framework, guides graduate students and clinicians in attaining practical skills for proposal planning and writing. Using a reflective-clinician approach, guidelines and checklists are provided to develop quality clinical project proposals. Students interact with the content through the ongoing reflective prompts and questions that guide them in reflective writing to better understand their projects and what they propose to do. The unique chapter format reminds students that development of a proposal is an integrative process, with many components that must be considered together. The following broad themes, corresponding to main sections of the book, organize the 16 chapters in a logical flow toward completion of planning and writing a clinical project proposal.

1. Writing Your Proposal: Putting Your "Problem" in Context. Putting a clinical problem in context, including an introduction to the topic and problem statement, is important in making the case for and outlining a project. Context also includes synthesizing the literature on a clinical topic and placing a project within that existing literature.

2. Writing Your Proposal: Designing and Setting the Stage for Your Project. The key points of a scholarly methods section that flows from a purpose statement are considered. Traditional quality improvement methods and research methods are discussed as tools for DNP projects.

3. Writing Your Proposal: Adding the Detail for Proposal Completion. The importance of visualizing the finished product; editing for concise, understandable language; and fine-tuning proposal methods and analyses are all considered. Next steps for using the project proposal are also considered.

This book provides students with tools to implement in their own scholarly practice. A chapter new to this edition focuses on quality-improvement concepts and provides the opportunity to further address this common approach to clinical projects. Chapters now feature boxes offering advice from doctor of nursing practice (DNP) students who have completed project proposals. New-project proposal abstracts have been added. Each chapter has been thoroughly updated and edited to enhance clarity. In response to reviewers' requests, websites for further learning have been added to most chapters. Key features to engage readers continue from the first edition; these include reflective questions, tips for making proposals complete and concise, exemplars, and reader activities. This text helps develop reflective clinical scholars who can write about clinical challenges, propose solutions, and use the methods of science to develop scholarly proposals.

Wanda Bonnel
Katharine V. Smith

Acknowledgments

The authors acknowledge the many individuals who have influenced the writing of this book. We thank our students, who continue to help us learn; our university colleagues for sharing ongoing discussions and ideas; and program graduates, who have shared resources for chapter examples. In addition, we thank our families for their ongoing encouragement and patience as we worked on this book. Thank you also to our Springer Publishing Company colleagues, especially Joseph Morita and Margaret Zuccarini, for encouragement through the development of this text.

Writing Your Proposal: Putting Your "Problem" in Context

Introduction: Why a Scholarly Proposal for the Clinical Project Proposal?

Reflective Questions

As you begin your work on a clinical project proposal, there are benefits to reflecting on your goals. You have ideas for the clinical project and are seeking further thoughts for turning these ideas into scholarly proposals that will lead to tight, strong, finished projects. The following reflective questions will help you consider your writing plan and organize learning for this chapter. Which of the following do you have the most comfort responding to?

- What makes a project proposal important?
- What does it mean to write a clinical project proposal?
- How do the concepts of *reflective clinician* and *clinical scholarship* relate?
- What makes a clinical proposal scholarly?
- How does best evidence fit with clinical projects?
- What are common terms related to best evidence and clinical project proposals?

• • •

PROPOSAL WRITING FOR SCHOLARLY CLINICAL PROJECTS: THE IMPORTANCE

This book is designed to help you become a reflective clinical scholar and to write proposals for clinical projects that impact patient care. Clinical scholarship is key to advancing patient care and at this time of change in health care, advanced clinical nursing scholarship is needed more than ever. Although a doctor of nursing practice (DNP) clinical project is designed to help improve patient care and safety for specific populations and systems, if carried out in a responsible way, strategies learned from this quality improvement project may also lead to a broader professional contribution that others might learn from. Your role in becoming a clinical scholar continues to increase as you learn to write proposals for clinical projects. Writing a clinical project proposal is one aspect of what you do as an advanced clinician as you plan a project that positively impacts your practice.

To write a clinical project proposal, one must have a design to follow. The concept of project design is key in proposal development. Design, as a broad concept, is often considered a tool for improvement. Designers can be considered agents of change. As an advanced clinician, you will be assessing current situations and in many cases proposing a change process for improving clinical outcomes. As proposal designer, the clinical project proposal can be one step in this development.

• • •

WRITING A CLINICAL PROJECT PROPOSAL

A proposal is a straightforward, logically organized, clear document that includes essential details that will guide a project. A proposal is considered the plan for how work will be designed to learn something important related to an interest area. Proposals are further described as a presentation of ideas; a study justification; and a work plan, which serves as evidence of a chain of reasoning, project feasibility, and a binding contract for proposed work (Krathwohl & Smith, 2005). The proposal plan needs to be logical, with the overall plan flowing from a problem statement. The proposal demonstrates how a need is met by this project and how it builds on previous work to address that need.

Scholarly clinical projects are one way you, as the advanced clinician, gain opportunities for making practice more visible to the public. Project aims can include promoting better patient care, supporting healthy people and community initiatives, and contributing to quality improvement in health care systems. The specific purpose of your clinical project may relate to addressing patient care outcomes that are about safety, quality care, quality of life, or patient transitions. As an advanced clinical practice nurse and leader, you develop clinical projects that integrate best evidence and consider contributions from other disciplines for the purpose of improving clinical practice.

The proposal is a written portion of the scholarly clinical project that "proposes" what is to be done to complete that project. It also situates the project within the existing literature on the topic. Once the proposal for the clinical project is approved, the clinical project is ready to be implemented. Once the proposed activities are completed, the proposal document then is adapted to become the final project summary. To complete the final summary paper, after the project is completed, the proposal methods section is changed to past tense (to show completion), and new sections on project results and implications are added. Thus, this proposal is a useful, versatile document that:

- Serves as a form of communication or as a type of information sharing
- Proposes what is to be done (provides the plan or proposed project outline to be implemented) so others can understand, provide approval, or even replicate it
- Identifies important, related literature
- Provides information in a written and scholarly format through which others can quickly find key concepts
- Serves as a type of contract identifying clear expectations for a class or program requirement
- Serves as the basis for becoming a final project document that integrates the project proposal and outcomes

This book guides you through steps for naming what you plan to do and describing to others how you plan to do it. For example, the Institute of Medicine (IOM; 2012) has identified the need for leadership in chronic care management. Advanced practice nurses have the opportunity to address population health issues to improve public health. Approaches, such as education and quality improvement, can be considered to help manage or control a chronic illness for a population subset. Designing a related clinical project could involve the following: naming a specific chronic illness and problem (such as osteoarthritis and pain management), selecting related concepts for further development or study that would lead to improved pain management (such as patient group coaching sessions on lifestyle modifications), reviewing the literature to determine the status of the evidence on the proposed concept, and finally framing this into a proposal for implementing or testing the best evidence to improve care of patients with osteoarthritis pain.

• • •

CLINICAL SCHOLARSHIP AND THE REFLECTIVE CLINICIAN

Clinical Scholarship

As recognized by the American Association of Colleges of Nursing (2015), all DNP students should implement a project that demonstrates clinical scholarship. Boyer (1990) described the importance of acknowledging clinical scholarship as well as sophisticated research programs. His classic framework for documenting scholarship includes frames of teaching, application, integration, and discovery. He provides a model for helping professionals not only share clinical products with others, but to reflect on and continue to improve these clinical products. Quality-improvement projects provide a good example of this process. Projects that serve as a type of quality improvement can help others know and learn from your observations and experiences. To meet the scholarship definition, components of product documentation, peer review, and publication or dissemination are required (Huber & Hutchings, 2005).

The Benefits of Reflection

Being an expert clinician or clinical leader comes with the responsibility of reflecting on practice issues to advance clinical patient care solutions. Reflection is a strategy that allows one to pause and think about what is going on; what is working or not working in a clinical or work-related situation. Reflection serves as a way to assess or identify gaps in clinical practice and move forward in clinical practice. Learning from these assessments often provides direction for future projects. As these ideas move to clinical project proposals, scholarly products and conversation that lead to clinical scholarship continue.

Critique of the current status of a particular care situation, for example, fall prevention, could involve addressing the problem from a systems perspective. This could incorporate reflection on the current unit or practice-site structures and processes (both needs and gaps) for gaining positive outcomes. Listening, observing, and writing about this situation provide a starting point for related project development. In this situation a reflective clinician asks: What is the team doing? How is it working? What could be better? These questions then lead to the opportunity for future clinical projects.

Scholarly writing is also related to reflection and scholarly dialogue; this scholarly dialogue involves reading the literature, communicating with others about that literature, and then developing your own scholarly proposal. Further reflection and scholarly dialogue occur with completed project proposals, implementation of the projects, and finally sharing this scholarship via the literature. Scholarly writing of proposals includes using methods of science and the language of the profession for disseminating the information contained in the clinical projects. Again, the scholarly proposal provides written communication to others. It communicates what you will do for the project and later it will be revised to communicate what you did. It provides the basis for a tight scholarly project that can be shared with others.

● ● ●

MAKING A CLINICAL PROPOSAL SCHOLARLY

Writing a scholarly proposal is part of a skill set needed to further clinical scholarship. Scholarly proposals provide a way to share, in a written and professional format, the important points of a major project. The proposal conveys not only what you will do, but why it is important that other people think about this topic. Your proposal summarizes your plans, provides a road map for implementing plans, and delivers to others a plan that they can review, critique, and approve. Scholarly proposals, and then completed projects, provide a means to contribute to the body of knowledge and improve clinical practice.

In your scholarly proposal you will use the language of science and a commonly accepted format for organizing project proposals and final papers. This consistency in structure promotes ease of communication within nursing and the larger, interdisciplinary community. The common sections for a scholarly proposal are:

- Introduction With Problem Summary and Purpose Statement
- Literature Review
- Project Methods

Although clinical project topics are quite variable, in all cases a proposal is an important component and serves as a project guide. In some ways completing a proposal is like putting together a puzzle and making sure all the pieces fit to give the best final picture. A scholarly proposal involves justifying and writing about your plan so that all of the clinical project pieces fit together.

Proposals serve as an important mechanism to clearly communicate about a proposed project. You will be communicating professionally in the literature and via conference presentations. Scholarly proposals incorporate the language of science with agreed-on terminology. Common agreement across disciplines dictates that scholarly proposals include clear presentation of problem summary, project purpose, literature review, project methods, and projected outcomes. Though this sounds simple, to make this happen there are numerous components to both consider and address. Although this book lays out components by chapter, it is important to consider the back-and-forth nature of each, for example, detailing the problem as a component of reviewing the literature. The art of scholarly proposing, in simple terms, includes:

- Starting with important problem
- Situating that problem in the literature and best evidence
- Framing it into a useful project, in writing, from which others can learn
- Making that written project proposal scholarly and doable

• • •

HOW DOES THE REFLECTIVE CLINICIAN USE EVIDENCE IN CLINICAL PROJECTS?

Scholarly dialogue includes reviewing best evidence in the literature as well as other professional sources of best evidence. Considering the state of the evidence can lead to further focus on the clinical problem. As you move forward in your proposal, you will begin asking questions that help you address how you will

- Further understand your concept
- Gain a process for evidence-based practice
- Enhance quality care
- Generate questions requiring further study

Once you have a beginning understanding of what is available in the literature or best evidence, then you are able to make decisions on the type of project that will be most needed related to your problem/topic. This allows you to focus broadly on using the evidence in advanced clinical projects such as the following:

- Synthesizing the literature on topics to develop current best-practice summaries or protocols for testing; an example would be sharing a synthesis of best evidence and protocols for promoting best anesthesia care for pediatric patients dealing with obesity
- Using and evaluating current best-evidence protocols to implement quality-improvement projects with unique populations; an example

would be teaching and evaluating use of an evidence-based protocol on diabetes management in long-term care settings
- Contributing to the evidence by sharing new clinical data; an example would be surveying rural advanced practice nurses related to their challenges and strategies for dealing with common rural-population issues

• • •

COMMON TERMS RELATED TO CLINICAL PROJECTS AND USE OF BEST EVIDENCE

Many terms and models exist to describe the process of best evidence for practice. Terms such as *translation of the evidence*, *research utilization*, and *evidence-based practice* can all relate to clinical projects and proposals. While a commonality in these terms includes synthesizing the evidence, there are unique components to each:

> *Translation of the evidence*: Translating evidence to knowledge for practice and helping staff become aware of and to access evidence-based resources
> *Research utilization*: Applying relevant studies to practice, after specific review and critique of each study
> *Evidence-based practice*: Expanding the concept of research utilization to include not only appropriate research in practice, but, when limited research evidence is available, other sources of best evidence, such as expert clinicians, are also considered; the patient preference for treatment is also a component

Also, the concepts of research, evaluation, and quality improvement are often discussed together. Again, there are similarities and differences in these basic terms, as well as frequent overlap of the concepts and methods used.

> *Evaluation*: Evaluative projects include systematic methods that judge the effectiveness of specific practices or policies.
> *Research*: Large-scale projects that involve systematic inquiry, using specified, disciplined methods of science in addressing problems or questions (Polit & Beck, 2012).
> *Quality improvement*: These projects analyze a system's performance and search for ways to improve quality using a formal approach with systematic methods (Duke University, 2005).

Relevant to these concepts, evaluation is a broad project approach/method used in both research and quality improvement. Research studies typically build in more controls to be more generalizable to other settings and populations. Quality improvement is typically considered narrower in focus and for specific institutional use.

• • •

CLINICAL SCHOLARSHIP: SEEKING AND GAINING A MENTOR

Seeking and gaining a mentor in the early stage of your work is an important and sometimes challenging task. Potential mentors should have expertise specific to content, settings, and methods. A mentor's availability, an interest in helping, and a strong commitment to your professional development are also important. The benefits of having a mentor are many, but, in particular, include helping you avoid pitfalls in determining feasibility or effectiveness of clinical project methods. When seeking a mentor, consider concepts of mutual readiness, opportunity, and resources for support. For example, if your mentor is at a distance, are methods available to facilitate conversations, and are both of you mutually interested in participating?

Finding a project mentor and using your project mentor(s) well is beneficial in all phases/aspects of project proposal development, as well as project implementation, evaluation, and completion. Consider the following strategies when seeking a mentor or to improve current work with a mentor:

- Focus on clear guidelines and expectations for both mentor and mentee
- Establish regular meeting times whether via phone, face to face, or in online meetings
- Find out when your mentor is available to read reports and what type of feedback your mentor is willing to give. Also ask about the lead time required to review documents.
- Build a schedule for project reports or updates
- Follow up on mentor's comments or suggestions
- If your mentor is at a distance, discuss electronic communication strategies

• • •

INTRODUCTION TO THE CLINICAL PROJECT TRIANGLE

As you move forward with your clinical project, you will want to consider the benefits of a clinical project triangle (Appendix A) and project checklist (Appendix B). The three points of the triangle include the project purpose, the methods, and the outcomes. This triangle helps hold the project together from a big-picture perspective and makes the project a cohesive whole. It is useful to begin a proposal with the triangle points in mind (subject to change as literature is reviewed and plans are finalized). For example, in a sample communications project, the purpose was seeking outcomes of improved communication between nursing staff and providers. Methods were then selected that could help achieve the designated outcomes. As noted, the purpose was broad and the methods and outcomes were quite specific. The goal is for all project points on the triangle to mesh so that all aspects of the project are consistent and the overall project is coherent.

Also learn from the experience of DNP students who have preceded you in the proposal-writing process. Their advice is presented in the following box.

• • •

ADVICE FROM DNP STUDENTS

Getting Started

Stay with it
- A project proposal needs to be a concise and clearly written paper that is easily transferrable.
- It all seems foreign at first, but once you start working through it a little bit at a time, and asking questions along the way, it starts to make sense.

Use the project triangle
- This triangle helps you to think through your project ideas and outline the work to be done.

SUMMARY

Clinicians have opportunities to impact patient care in health care systems that are changing. Being an expert clinician or clinical leader comes with the responsibility of reflecting on practice issues and advancing clinical patient care solutions via scholarly projects. Clinical project proposals provide a way to begin naming the areas you would like to effect. Proposals for clinical projects directed at solving clinical problems can be implemented and shared as a form of scholarly practice.

TIPS FOR GETTING STARTED

As you begin your clinical project, here are some tips to help you:

- Schedule regular times to reflect on a problem topic of interest for your project. Initially avoid getting bogged down in detail. Note and relate facts, your reactions and feelings, and note both frustrations and "aha" moments (Zachary, 2000).
- Add something to your reflections at each scheduled work session. Even if you are not productive at first, this establishes the routine and sets the expectation to help you develop a regular work pattern.
- Prepare to address the questions your reflections raise: What is the evidence on this topic of interest? What is the state of current practice in a specified location or population? What value is there in further addressing this problem?

WEBSITES FOR FURTHER REVIEW

Although this text is designed to help with a variety of clinical projects, broad guides that provide background on DNP projects can be found on websites of select national organizations. Examples are:

- *The Doctor of Nursing Practice: Current Issues and Clarifying Recommendations (AACN):*
  www.aacn.nche.edu/aacn-publications/white-papers/DNP-Implementation-TF-Report-8-15.pdf
- *The Doctorate of Nursing Practice NP Preparation: NONPF Perspective 2015:*
  c.ymcdn.com/sites/www.nonpf.org/resource/resmgr/DNP/NONPFDNPStatementSept2015.pdf
- *Defining Scholarship for the Discipline of Nursing:*
  www.aacn.nche.edu/publications/position/defining-scholarship

NEXT CHAPTER UP

Chapter 2 provides practical guides for getting started with your writing plan. The chapter addresses gaining ideas and tips for writing, asking the right questions, and making good choices to craft project proposals.

LEARNING ACTIVITIES

Beginning Writing Prompts

Writing prompts provide a way to reflect and get some ideas on paper. Use these prompts to brainstorm possibilities.

- Some of the big concerns I have with my clinical work relate to . . .
- If there is one clinical or work-related problem I would fix, it would be . . . and the outcomes I would be interested in would include . . .
- The people and place factors that impact this problem are . . .
- If I could focus on just one aspect of this problem, it would be . . .

Writing an Initial Reflection

Begin a written reflection by sharing what has shaped your ideas about a specific topic/problem. What have been your experiences or lessons learned? Then consider how these might be similar or different from others' perspectives.

* COVID-19 and how it has affected the patient's Mental & physical health needs

→ PHQ/GAD Screens & Survey for Symptoms experienced

→ Trial medication/download Apps educational handouts

→ ✓ and assess effectiveness after usage of meds/apps/handouts

→ Screening for mental health issues in Primary Care during the pandemic: A QI project

Checklist and Goal Setting: Readiness to Begin a Clinical Project

On a scale of 1 (low) to 3 (high), how would you rate yourself on each of the following points? What further goals need to be addressed?

At this point in time . . .

- I am motivated to help improve patient outcomes via advanced clinical projects.
- I have beginning clinical challenges/ideas I would like to further develop.
- I am in a situation that supports moving forward with a clinical project.
- I am ready to communicate professionally via a written proposal.

REFERENCES

American Association of Colleges of Nursing Task Force on the Implementation of the DNP. (2015, August). The doctor of nursing practice: Current issues and clarifying recommendations. Retrieved from http://www.aacn.nche.edu/news/articles/2015/dnp-white-paper

Boyer, E. L. (1990). *Scholarship reconsidered: Priorities of the professoriate.* Princeton, NJ: Carnegie Foundation for the Advancement of Teaching.

Duke University. (2005). Patient safety—Quality improvement. Retrieved from http://patientsafetyed.duhs.duke.edu/index.html

Huber, M., & Hutchings, P. (2005). The advancement of learning: Building the teaching commons. San Francisco, CA: Jossey-Bass.

Institute of Medicine. (2012). *Living well with chronic illness: A call for public health action.* Washington, DC: National Academies Press.

Krathwohl, D., & Smith, N. (2005). *How to prepare a dissertation proposal: Suggestions for students in education and the social and behavioral sciences.* Syracuse, NY: Syracuse University Press.

Polit, D., & Beck, C. T. (2012). *Nursing research generating and assessing evidence for nursing practice* (9th ed.). Baltimore, MD: Lippincott Williams & Wilkins.

Zachary, L. J. (2000). *The mentor's guide: Facilitating effective learning relationships.* San Francisco, CA: Jossey-Bass.

2

...

Using the Writing Plan as a Developmental Tool for the Advanced Clinical Project

Reflective Questions

Clearly written communication is a powerful tool in health care. Its presence is credited with avoiding system errors and promoting quality care. In Chapter 1 your focus was thinking about what you do as a clinician and beginning to identify where clinical improvements are needed for a project. You considered the importance of your scholarly project proposal. In this chapter you begin to address the clear writing that is essential in the proposal; each section within the proposal has specific needs and guidelines to comply with standards of scholarly writing. The following reflective questions organize learning for this chapter. With which of the following are you the most comfortable?

- Why is this writing plan important? What makes clinical scholarship and proposal writing go together?
- What does it mean to organize and draft a writing plan? Why a self-directed learning and writing focus?
- What are strategies to begin and to keep the scholarly writing plans moving forward?

A good clinical project, written first as a clinical proposal, guides and enhances project quality for credible outcomes. Reflective clinicians begin a proposal by seeing a problem, generating a plan for dealing with the problem through the proposal process, and then implementing the proposed clinical project. Reflective clinicians, as self-directed writers, follow steps that guide the proposal write-up, taking ideas and meshing them with project guidelines or templates for quality projects.

A written proposal is the first formal step of a clinical project and is a form of clinical scholarship. This chapter is about organizing and getting started with the writing plan. It is also about being a reflective clinician and sharing through writing. This chapter moves you forward in considering reading and writing together, gaining a plan for self-directed writing, drafting a scholarly writing plan, and strategies to use to keep the scholarly writing process moving along.

● ● ●

CONSIDERING SCHOLARLY WRITING AND READING TOGETHER

Writing as a Tool in Considering a Good Problem and Project Approaches

The goal is to write a proposal that clearly names your project plans. This accomplishes three things: (a) it allows you to clarify what you will be doing in your project, (b) it helps others understand the intent of the project, and (c) it provides a map or guide so that others can understand the merit of the project and replicate the project in other settings. You can begin drafting a plan by answering these questions: Who am I writing for? Who is my audience? What are the rules? As you name and learn about specific clinical issues of interest, you are reflecting and writing about them.

Linking Scholarly Writing With Reading

At this stage in the clinical project, reading and writing fit together. While reading, you are gaining a big picture of the topic and planning how to situate your specific issue within its appropriate context (including both its setting and available literature in the area). This involves gaining an orientation to your topic and evidence-based resources.

- Use active reading to narrow the field (preview articles and consider questions to address further in reading)
- As you read, develop questions about studies and findings: who, what, where, how large, and how outcomes are gained

Typically, you have focused on reading to learn more about specific practice concepts. At this point you are also reading to consider approaches that might be used to help move your clinical project forward. What do you learn from what others have done that can be used to package projects in meaningful ways that could benefit colleagues, staff, and students?

• • •

A PLAN FOR SELF-DIRECTED WRITING: PREWRITING AND THE BROAD WRITING PLAN

Why should you care about the writing plan? Because a limited plan typically means a limited product. Because you have limited hours, you have to maximize your use of those hours. The writing plan is important because it helps outline the important points and makes writing a central tool. Just as planning in nursing is central to patient care, the larger clinical project can be considered to take a similar "care plan" approach in assessing project need, clearly stating the problem, outlining possible approaches, and then selecting the best of each for the situation. This includes evaluation used to determine how the project plan is working.

Prewriting

Prewriting occurs before official proposal writing starts. This refers to the point at which you get organized and ready to write. It can include getting yourself to your writing place; sticking to the time you have allotted; having a beverage in hand; and getting sufficient reading, thinking, and exploring done to lead your writing down the right path (putting together reading notes that can later be cited is also useful).

Prewriting also provides an opportunity for early organization of thoughts or to clarify problems, as well as to help identify what your project is *not* about (Wolcott, 2008). Because this prewriting helps focus your ideas, the project becomes more reasonable and then becomes a more doable project. Your actual problem can become clearer through this process. It provides opportunities to consider other phases of the work.

Sometimes reflecting on broad questions serves as a good prewriting tool. For example, why is this topic interesting to me? Specific writing tools, such as project decision trails or reflective journals, help you document your work, the acts of reflecting and journaling help assess what is working or not with your project plans. Writing and critical thinking make a good connection.

Getting-started tips for organizing a writing plan, including your writing time and space, consist of:

- When to write? When thinking about your time organization, does your plan involve a calendar/a clock? Are you a morning or night person? What's compatible with your personal and family life?
- Where to write? Your writing space counts, too. Do you require a quiet, peaceful place to write or can you write anywhere? Often selecting one central writing area, with organized supplies and resources, helps writing efficiency. An added bonus is finding a spot where you can spread out and not have to pick up every time after you have finished working.
- What to write? Anything; just start to get something on paper. Then work into the specific proposal components you are addressing.

Tips to Maintain Momentum for Your Writing Plan

Many life events will distract you from writing. Try to put writing first for selected time periods (other than emergencies). Tips for keeping momentum include:

- Develop a big-picture project map that helps you stay on track
- Be realistic in goal setting or doability of plans; describe deliverables
- Organize tasks with a timeline and check it regularly
- Be clear and enthusiastic about goals
- Identify a mentor or colleague as a support person
- Identify someone besides yourself to whom you're responsible for accomplishing specified work and meeting due dates

● ● ●

DRAFTING THE SCHOLARLY WRITING PLAN

Organization is important and different for scholarly proposals than it is for other types of writing. Although textbooks are written for broad audiences to highlight and summarize key content areas, in a clinical proposal the format becomes more prescriptive. For example, at least three focused sections are addressed in scholarly proposals, including (a) the introduction (with problem summary and project purpose statement); (b) literature review and synthesis; and (c) methods. Specific sections, such as the methods section, then address further project components (project design, sample, data collection, and data-analysis plans). Future chapters will elaborate these topics.

To begin organizing the scholarly writing plan, reflective questions and written responses can help make the connections to puzzling problems. Sample questions include:

- *What will you be doing?* When writing the scholarly proposal, there are multiple concepts to consider. This will include addressing what is known about your problem or clinical project topic and including the literature review (what others have written on the subject). You will also be explaining the plan for your project.
- *Who will you be writing for?* There are different rules/guidelines for different audiences. Are you writing for a clinical project committee? A research review board? A course faculty member? Who else are you writing this proposal for? Spend time considering your various audiences and the implications of these different groups for the project proposal expectations and requirements.
- *What tools/techniques are available?* It's important to know about the available resources for increasing efficiency as well as effectiveness. In addition to the broad proposal guidelines outlined in this text, often specific guidelines are available to assist you in crafting clinical project proposals with specific purposes such as coursework or grant funding. To begin, what specific guidelines are available to guide you in crafting the proposal? Are there templates to guide completion? Is there a time frame for proposal completion? Is there a page limit? From a practical perspective, drafting an early table of contents that outlines all the required components is a useful strategy.
- *What are your qualifications?* What education and experiences have prepared you to propose and write up a specific project proposal? Or to use specific methods? Or to even study the proposed concept? Just as an athlete would not undertake a major athletic event without preparing, it is important that you also have or gain the background, education, and skills to propose and complete the clinical project.
- *Are there practical concerns or ethical issues in a particular topic?* As part of clinical projects, both practical and ethical issues and concerns must be addressed. For example, if you would like to learn more about patient function in specific home settings for your elderly population, what practical issues must be addressed in making home visits? What potential ethical issues might need to be addressed if you wanted to take videos of the patient in the home for analysis?

- *Will you be able to carry out the project you are proposing?* Striving for a project that is not too big and not too small can be a challenge when you first begin your project planning. Mentor and peer review can provide the benefit of additional perspectives to help deal with finding the proper balance.

● ● ●

STRATEGIES TO KEEP THE SCHOLARLY WRITING PLAN MOVING FORWARD

Motivation for doing clinical projects is often high while thinking and planning, but students anecdotally share that actually writing the proposal can be a challenge. Considering the proposal from the positive frame of thinking through the "big picture" and keeping the end result in mind can be a form of motivation. Writing the proposal with the project triangle in mind, with the goal to ultimately getting the purpose, methods, and outcomes in alignment, will provide the foundation for a well-organized clinical project that helps improve clinical practice.

Big-Picture Tools and Problem-Solving Strategies

All scholarly writers need a good starting point and tools to keep moving their writing forward. Starting with a good clinical problem (Chapter 3) can help motivate you and keep you moving forward. For example, finding an area of interest or a concern/challenge (that you believe will truly improve patient care) and then studying it with a quick assessment of related concepts/issues through a concept map can be helpful. Concept maps have the benefit of visualizing multiple related concepts or issues that may be related to or influencing the problem.

Problem solving fits with concept mapping as a brainstorming tool to identify possible antecedents to the problem and to identify particular patterns that emerge. Visualize or push your thinking first to the big picture of the problem and then to the full project.

Other tools to visualize big-picture issues include diagramming and outlining approaches. These have the benefit of exposing the big picture of potential aggravating or causative factors. As noted, using a fishbone-type diagram can help identify important factors or components influencing problems. Additional approaches, such as problem-solving question prompts, can help one brainstorm. Brainstorming, or rapidly generating ideas relevant to your topic, is valuable as you begin a project. This includes asking the right questions such as: What if? and I wonder . . .? Paragraphs highlighting sample planning tools are presented here.

Mind Mapping or Concept Mapping

Mind mapping and concept mapping tools provide a visual approach to help name your problem and its context. Developing concept maps provides a beginning reflective activity. Maps help you think about key points surrounding a particular problem and provide potential options to consider before making your case as to why this is an important problem. These visual approaches might also help as you seek themes from your literature review. When completed after a literature review, these can also help you determine what evidence there is (or needs to be gained) to make your case. Moving beyond basic concept identification, further diagramming can help identify possible interrelations (such as spider diagrams or extended Venn diagrams). Asking who, what, when, and where can also help diagram the topic/plan.

Planning Arrows

With similarities to concept maps, planning arrows help organize thinking on specific topics. Sometimes called a *fishbone diagram*, this tool provides direction in naming potential challenges impacting one problem area. Using a systems perspective, planning arrows remind you to consider structure-and-process issues that may be impacting particular topics and outcomes.

Reflective Writing Strategies

Reflection provides an opportunity for making sense of experiences and can lead to quality-improvement opportunities (Kaplan, Silver, LaVaque-Manty, & Meizlish, 2013; Sherwood & Horton-Deutsch, 2012). Reflection is a key tool to use not only to begin writing, but also to keep writing progressing. Reflection, along with scholarly dialogue and writing projects, is a tool that can also help evaluate clinical challenges, generate further questions, and potentially lead to problem solutions. Reflecting and generating further questions go hand in hand. Reflective responses to questions can help focus and stimulate thinking, encouraging new thoughts and responses to challenges.

The One-Page Early Reflection

One approach to using reflection as you begin a project is to start by writing about why you are choosing a particular topic. This would include, for example, the interests that led you to this topic. If you have several topics in mind, complete a one-page reflective paper on each topic that addresses the following: What do I already know/think/feel about this topic? What questions do I still have? These reflections help address why these topics/projects are important to you and which will be the most interesting and provide the greatest clinical value to you and others. Other reflective-writing techniques can be helpful at various points in the project.

Ongoing Reflective Journaling

Ongoing journaling, spending even 10 to 15 minutes a day on a project, can promote success. It is important just to establish the writing routine or habit and get something project related on paper. For a jump start, combine this habit with already established rituals, such as a morning cup of coffee.

- *The concept of structured questions or writing prompts* to guide written reflections adds more direction to journaling. This practice promotes tracking what you already know about your project and helps identify areas needing further attention or further inquiry (Wolcott, 2008). Consider using the reflective questions incorporated throughout this text as writing prompts to get you going and keep you going.
- *Free writing* leads to learning more about your thoughts and subsequently organizing those thoughts. Free writing involves letting words flow without concern for spelling, edits, or others' eyes. The goal is to simply get content/thoughts on paper. You then have something to edit and share with colleagues that conveys your thoughts for further discussion.

Tools to Help Document and Further the Writing Plan

Especially when writing a large project over time, there are benefits to outlining and record-keeping tools that help track factual information, resources, and project decisions.

Outlining is described as an art and offers the following benefits: firms up thinking, organizes materials, and gains a logical step-by-step method. Providing a type of visual impression, an outline can help identify gaps or excesses in writing plans, promoting unity and emphasis on key points (Savers, 2011). Although some prefer a detailed outline as part of the writing plan, others use a broad outline format, focusing only on broad concepts that will guide, rather than focusing on numbered details. Experiment with both and see which is more helpful to you.

Decision trails or *decision logs* are factual records. They include keeping an annotated list of your work and decisions as you go along. This provides a record of what actually has been done and also can help you remember why you made the decisions you did, serving as a type of summary. It allows you to keep track of processes undertaken and ongoing challenges as well as accomplishments.

* * *

SEEKING WRITING REVIEWS WITH THE PROJECT TEAM

Communicating With the Project Team

It is important to maintain clear dialogue with project mentors and other team members, as well as written follow-up communications. In communicating with your project mentor or other team members, have an agenda for your meeting. This includes a list of specific questions you would like to discuss. Listen actively to gain the other person's viewpoint.

Send follow-up communication to confirm clear and consistent understanding on both parts. Share, for example, "This is what I heard at our meeting and these are the points I will follow-up on." When you are asked to make revisions, make sure you show on your follow-up document where those changes were made (e.g., using different text color or the Track Changes feature in Word).

Self-Editing

You will want to start with self-editing, a process in which you read and reread your written work to make sure it clearly states your intended ideas. As the number of times you read your own words increases, it's easy to start gliding over them too quickly to edit effectively, so it's helpful to read your work out loud to slow yourself down and to hear different inflections that can be read into your wording and punctuation choices. It is particularly useful to evaluate your work against an available proposal rubric. This step often helps avoid missing important proposal components. Also putting the paper aside and then revisiting it after several days provides an opportunity for clearer self-evaluation of the writing.

Peer and Mentor Reviews

Peer and mentor reviews are also good editing approaches. Peer review includes reviewing, interpreting, and communicating evaluative information to a colleague. This can be a formal or informal process that helps nurses provide feedback to peers based on specific criteria. Typically, this is an interactive process and involves use of specified guidelines or rubrics based on criteria to guide the feedback. Remember that a combination of positive and constructive feedback is most helpful—exclusively positive feedback feels good and exclusively negative feedback is destructive, and neither contributes to excellence; hence, be sure to provide a balance between positive and constructive comments.

Seeking formal reviews from mentors is also key. Points to consider include:

- Be proactive in seeking/gaining feedback on your writing trouble spots.
- If you note trouble spots in your writing, rework what you have written. If you cannot give up any of your initial paragraph drafts, open a file named "Extra" to copy and paste information for potential future use.
- Seek out writing centers at schools or from private resources to guide you if you are experiencing problems conveying your thoughts clearly. Writing centers provide guidance, not on your content, but on your process for organizing and conveying written information.

Also learn from the experience of DNP students who have preceded you in the proposal-writing process. Their advice is presented in the following box.

• • •

ADVICE FROM DNP STUDENTS

Beginning to Write Your Proposal

Make sure you know the proposal guidelines
- Clearly identify expectations and additional resources to assist you in proposal development.

Think about your proposal in sections (similar to scholarly articles)
- Try to go step by step. The various steps need to be considered in a systematic way to organize and develop a successful project.
- It helps to know how to "talk the research language."

Use an outline to help know ahead of time what you will be writing
- Think about the process (or parts/sections) for pulling together the parts of a DNP proposal.

(continued)

* Clearly outline the methods section. It is extremely helpful to do the outline first. This facilitates writing.

Focus on reflection
* It helps to constantly reflect on where you are. When you get stuck, go back to the project questions and reflect; it helps.

SUMMARY

Although much of this chapter focuses on approaches to writing a clinical project, it is also about tools that make writing a part of clinical scholarship. Writing is a way to name and package what you are doing or planning to do. A writing plan can lead to successful proposals that then lead to successful clinical projects. The self-directed writer becomes adept at organizing time, place, and space. There are various tools to help the clinician writer stay motivated and organized to move forward with writing tasks for clinical projects.

TIPS FOR GETTING STARTED

As you begin your writing, here are some tips to help you:

* Stay focused on the project topic.
* Get something written down.
* Gain writing experience.
* Address the beginnings–middles–endings formula, like "speech" class, to help you outline a proposal section. In addition to the main "middle" message, the introduction summarizes what you will tell the reader and why it is important. An effective conclusion then summarizes what has been accomplished.
* Use time-management strategies like tracking the time allotted and used for clinical proposal writing.
* Remember your decision trail and journaling to record your ideas/ decisions.

WEBSITES FOR FURTHER REVEIW

Writing practice, or "just writing," can be valuable in developing a clear proposal. Strategies for supporting writing plans (both informal and formal) can be found in select websites. Examples are:

- *Clear Communication Messages* (a toolkit for communications skills from MindTools):
  www.mindtools.com/pages/main/communication_skills.htm
- *How to Write a Paragraph: The Art of Substantive Writing* (full book reference):
  www.criticalthinking.org/store/get_file.php?inventories_id=160
- *The Aspiring Thinker's Guide to Critical Thinking*:
  www.criticalthinking.org/files/SAM_Aspiring_Thinkers_GuideOPT.pdf

NEXT CHAPTER UP

How do you shape the problem statement? You have ideas, a plan for writing; now it is time to focus on organizing information on one specific problem area. Moving from the messy "problem" to the real issue and fine-tuned problem statement is a next step.

LEARNING ACTIVITIES

Writing Prompts

Writing prompts provide a way to reflect and get some ideas written down. Use these prompts to brainstorm possibilities.

- I want to study more about this topic because . . .
- My background will help in the following ways . . .
- Areas I still need to gain knowledge/skill in include . . .
- A beginning plan for gaining these skills includes . . .

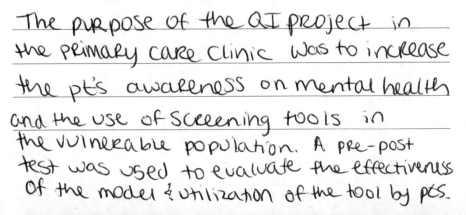

The purpose of the QI project in the primary care clinic was to increase the pt's awareness on mental health and the use of screening tools in the vulnerable population. A pre-post test was used to evaluate the effectiveness of the model & utilization of the tool by pts.

Checklist and Goal Setting for Generating a Writing Plan

To which of the following can you check "yes"? Which of the following needs to be further addressed?

Are you:

- Writing regularly with reasonable ease?
- Focusing on what you are to be writing?
- Avoiding distractions of excess reading/other?
- Using peers/advisors when needed?
- Using an efficient writing process?
- Moving forward?

Do you:

- Have a project/writing timetable?
- Feel good about your writing process?
- Have a process that's working for you?
- Have a steady writing pace that feels reasonable?
- Have a pace consistent with your calendar for finishing the project (Bolker, 1998)?

REFERENCES

Bolker, J. (1998). *Writing your dissertation in fifteen minutes a day: A guide to starting, revising, and finishing your doctoral thesis*. Brighton, Victoria, Australia: Owl Publishing.

Kaplan, M., Silver, N., LaVaque-Manty, D., & Meizlish, D. (2013). *Using reflection and metacognition to improve student learning: Across the disciplines, across the academy*. Sterling, VA: Stylus Book.

Savers, C. (2011). *Anatomy of writing for publication for nurses*. Indianapolis, IN: Sigma Theta Tau International.

Sherwood, G., & Horton-Deutsch, S. (2012). *Reflective practice: Transforming education and improving outcomes*. Indianapolis, IN: Sigma Theta Tau International.

Wolcott, H. (2008). *Writing up qualitative research*. Thousand Oaks, CA: Sage.

3

Writing a Good Clinical Problem Statement and Placing the Clinical Problem in Context

Reflective Questions

In Chapter 2, you learned about tips for organizing your writing. Now the focus is on determining and naming the problem that will be the subject of your writing, putting that problem in context, and creating a written problem statement. The following reflective questions organize learning for this chapter. With which of the following are you the most comfortable?

- Identifying areas of clinical practice that you find most interesting, problematic, alarming, or confusing?
- Isolating problematic areas of clinical practice that could be changed to improve patient care?
- Clarifying the problem name and its description/definition?
- Explaining the significance of finding a solution to the problem?

• • •

FROM AREA OF CONCERN TO PROBLEM STATEMENT

This chapter is about taking an area of concern and turning it into a clearly named problem. Broadly described, clinical problems relate to topics that provide clinicians and clinical leaders opportunities to improve patient care. A problem refers to a situation that needs a solution. Naming a problem can lead to evaluating and packaging new approaches that promote safe clinical care delivery and products for clinical education and leadership. Good problems have good practical implications, are well delineated, and promote personal and career interests (Krathwohl & Smith, 2005). The final problem statement sets the stage for generating the project purpose and methods for completing the work.

Where Do Areas of Concern or Problems Come From?

As you know, clinical problems come in all shapes and sizes. As a good reflective clinician, you probably have many "problem" ideas already. Current nursing specialty problems or "issues" that may serve as project ideas are often described via professional nursing meetings, funding sources, and specialty newsletters. It is also important to look around and see what current challenges exist in your clinical setting. What is happening, or not happening, that impacts safe, quality care? Sometimes this problem is approached using a gap analysis, the space between "what is and what should be." In other words, what still needs to happen related to the area of concern?

Clinical problems can be unique or common. Some will have relevance to specific areas of a unique practice setting. Others might have relevance to diverse settings or broad health-promotion issues of populations. Sample brainstorming options to help you generate specific clinical problem areas include:

- Wondering about clinical unit problems from recent practice experiences uncovered any clinical unit problems? Is there a better way? Could what worked well in one setting be considered in your current setting? For example, wondering if a specific evidence-based communication protocol would enhance your own unit communication.
- Having conversations with others and reviewing competence in clinical practice settings. Are staff demonstrating current clinical competencies that match current national standards? What practice concerns do your colleagues identify?
- Thinking about ways to improve staff education on clinical topics, documentation standards, or interprofessional practices. For example, are current pain-management protocols expanded to include holistic healing approaches?
- Considering clinical needs for quality improvement (QI). Ask, for example, whether best policies and practices are being used in select areas such as peripherally inserted central catheter (PICC) line practices.

In this chapter, as part of thinking about a problem area that you want to focus on for your clinical project, several "problem" aspects are considered. For example, how do you focus a problem for study? How do you know it is an important problem that needs to be addressed in your setting, and how do you know that you are choosing a reasonable problem to pursue as a scholarly clinical project? More specific needs assessments for addressing a particular issue are addressed in future chapters.

• • •

FOCUSING THE PROBLEM: BRINGING IDEAS INTO SHAPE

The goal is to take a broad problem area, or area of concern, and turn it first into a focused problem and then a specific problem statement, moving from a general problem to a specific problem. Areas of concern are different from focused problems. Areas of concern typically involve numerous broad interacting issues rather than a detailed focused problem. For example, as a clinical leader in long-term care, naming the group dining setting for frail elders as a "mess" may accurately state an area of concern, but it lacks direction for improving the elders' dining situation. Moving from a broad, fuzzy area of concern to a specific problem(s) is one of the first parts of project development. What do you specifically mean by your "problem"? In this group dining situation, are there staffing issues? A lack of adaptive equipment? Poor environmental arrangements?

When you have identified a broad area of concern, consider whether any of the additional brainstorming tools could be used to further focus the problem. Brainstorming tools can help first identify big-picture issues (e.g., the top of a funnel), but they can also help in narrowing to a more specific aspect of a broad problem. These tools can also help clearly name what the problem or issue is and what the surrounding factors are. Additional strategies to use to help clarify the problem and to consider a problem's context include:

- Root-cause analyses or fishbone diagrams, which help name and organize the potential factors that can be impacting a problem
- Concept maps or concentric-circle diagrams
- Addressing the who, what, why, where, and when related to a particular problem, which can also help focus a problem

Again, early project work involves making sure you are identifying and naming a problem that can be focused. Once the problem is named, then you will go on to write a problem statement and then, following that, you will write the project purpose statement. Concurrent with this writing process, you will be searching the literature. The literature review adds to finding out what is known and not known about this clinical problem in the profession. It addresses whether and/or how others have considered or addressed this or similar problems.

The literature related to your area of concern not only helps with naming and describing the problem of interest, but can also help as you move forward in thinking about a potential project plan. The literature review helps you identify if there are numerous scholarly publications on the topic, suggesting that your problem topic is evidence rich, or conversely that there are few publications with limited evidence related to your topic. It addresses whether the evidence you are finding can help with further solution planning. For example, as you have conversations with other professionals about the group dining room in your long-term care setting, your use of problem-solving models and review of the literature can help identify various issues that lead to problems within this setting.

Sample approaches used to gain ideas on topics of interest or problem areas include:

- Reading broadly and then becoming more specialized
- Reviewing tables of contents for sample naming of problems or approaches to a problem
- Reviewing textbooks on a topic of interest to identify broad challenges
- Seeking synthesis articles first and then following up with specific studies
- Contacting experts in the field

• • •
_____

FOCUSING THE PROBLEM: NARROWING THE TOPIC

Once you begin describing the problem, there is almost always benefit to narrowing your topic to be very specific for your project. This helps in naming the problem more clearly, guiding the literature review, and then projecting further clinical study plans. In essence you are seeking movement from that fuzzy area of concern or "mess" to a clear problem statement and potential plan. Narrowing or funneling, seeing the change from a large global problem to a more concrete, detailed problem, helps focus the problem to a more doable clinical project topic. A funneling method, starting broadly and then narrowing the options, is done by continuing to ask whether a more narrow focus will help name this problem or issue more clearly, as well as lead to a more focused useful study approach.

For example, related to the group dining topic in long-term care, thoughts might proceed as follows: the group dining room situation is a "mess" and needs to function better; then asking, which patient groups are having the most challenges? Then, what does the literature say about working with these patient groups? Or perhaps you will determine another pathway to narrow the problem, such as staffing issues that seem to be problematic; then, which staff seem to have the most challenges helping patients or who could provide more help? What does the literature say about staffing issues, both in general and in long-term care dining settings?

Using another example, even if you have determined there is a unit need for palliative care education, you still have a very broad statement with limited specifics about what that means. Moving forward you would take this broad topic and determine specific educational areas for your focus. Looking at this broad topic, sample approaches might be to narrow it to areas such as pain or symptom management or family involvement in care. These concepts could be further explored and narrowed to the many areas, all within this broad problem, that could help improve patient care. When a range of options is identified, it becomes easier to focus on the specific needs for unit staff education and to further focus a project plan. As noted in the palliative care education example, most problems start broad and then need to be narrowed to a much more specific, direct focus. Once you have narrowed the focus, it will be easier to move forward in naming and packaging what you will do in your clinical project.

• • •

FOCUSING THE PROBLEM: CLARIFYING THE PROBLEM NAME AND DESCRIPTION

Why is clarifying the problem name important? Basically you have to make sure that your project team and future readers know what you mean by the use of the selected term. You will have to confirm that others agree with this terminology or that your use of the term is consistent with how others (e.g., in the literature) are using it. Even if your project becomes a broad exploratory approach to learn more about the problem, you will still need broad descriptors of the concept you are studying. Depending on the problem you choose to study, describing/defining is often considered similar to or a basic step of concept analysis, which is discussed in Chapter 6. Resources, such as the work of Walker and Avant (2011), provide further details.

For example, if you are concerned about the problem of increasing incidents of delirium in health care settings, first you will need to define and describe what is meant by *delirium*. How does the best evidence or literature define and use the term? If you wish to pursue a project that includes palliative care education, you will need to further define what the term *palliative care* means, for example, differentiating or identifying similarities and differences to the concept of hospice. Note also that you have indicated the concept of education as a part of the problem solution. For a scholarly project you need to further describe what the concept of education will mean. The basic question to address is: What are you naming your concepts and how are you defining your concepts for study? That includes naming what the concepts are as well as clarifying what they are not.

• • •

FOCUSING THE PROBLEM: DESCRIBING CONTEXT AND SETTING BOUNDARIES

What makes the problem context and problem boundaries important considerations? Part of naming and defining the problem includes putting the chosen problem in a selected setting and identifying the problem boundaries for purposes of the project. Context is the broad setting, and the boundaries establish what is included in and excluded from that context.

Describing the context of a project includes helping others better understand the people, place, and process factors related to your project. Providing the right amount of detail (e.g., describing that the project is set in an emergency room in a small rural hospital versus a large urban medical center) helps others understand your project context. This will be particularly useful to others in helping to determine whether a similar project might work in their settings.

Naming or setting the boundaries helps you and your reader understand what you are doing, as well as what are you not doing, related to this problem. Stating, for example, that "x" will be included in the project but "y" will not helps identify the boundaries of the problem you plan to study and frames the problem to more clearly identify where it stops and starts. This also helps limit the extraneous issues and extraneous data, making the project more clear and manageable. For example, which of the following provides more focus?

- The context/boundaries for this project are all elderly patients in this hospital with risk factors for delirium.
- The context/boundaries for this project are patients with a dementia diagnosis on a specific surgical unit who are at risk for delirium.

Note that the second statement provides more direction. The intent is to further narrow and determine what is most important and most feasible or practical to include in the project (Leedy & Omrod, 2013). In simple terms, this means putting a frame or boundary around the topic/problem/issue you are addressing and then describing the surrounding factors. The Standards for Quality Improvement Reporting Excellence (SQUIRE; 2015) resources provide additional discussion about this topic.

* * *

WHAT MAKES THIS A GOOD AND IMPORTANT PROBLEM TO STUDY?

What makes your problem an important one to study? Why is this problem significant to others? Does it matter or make a contribution to practice? Does it address a practical, clinical concern? Use the following additional questions (Leedy & Omrod, 2013) to guide your thinking during problem-statement development and write-up.

1. Is the problem of current interest? Is it topical?
2. Is the problem likely to continue into the future?
3. Will more information about the problem have practical or theoretical applications?
4. How large is the population affected by the problem?
5. How would study of this problem lead to improving the problem or extend existing knowledge about the problem?
6. Would clinical project findings potentially lead to some useful change in best practice?
7. Is there current research or evidence that supports the need for further study of this problem?

* * *

INTRODUCING THE PROBLEM IN THE PROPOSAL

Problem Significance

Discussion of the problem significance provides the rationale for why you are taking on the project. Much of the challenge is articulating the specific clinical problems and challenges so that others understand. Here you introduce and make the case for the importance of the problem you want to address. This includes describing the background of the problem. Addressing broad issues includes providing a brief summary of current knowledge of the problem being addressed in broad populations or organizations. Addressing local issues includes describing the nature and severity of the specific local problem or system dysfunction to be addressed. Finally, summarize a specific statement of the problem to be addressed in the project. This problem statement then leads to identifying the project purpose, setting the stage for determining best methods to guide the project.

Fine-Tuning the Problem Statement

The problem statement serves to describe the important issues or conditions that exist in leading to the proposed project. An effective problem statement names the extent of the problem and supporting evidence, identifies factors contributing to the situation, and notes current gaps in addressing the problem (Coley & Scheinberg, 2007).

Although the background of the problem is described in multiple paragraphs, a specific statement comprised of several sentences that summarizes the problem is beneficial to you in clearly naming the problem as well as communicating its significance to others. This statement clearly identifies your area of concern as a specific problem and provides the focused name of an issue you plan to study in some way. It names what the problem is and clarifies what it is not. The problem statement is part of the first section of the proposal and introduces the reader to your problem. After reading your summary of the problem, ask yourself:

- Can I clearly answer the question: "What is the problem"?
- Is the scope appropriately limited with a balance of completeness and conciseness?
- Can I state why this problem is important and why it is worthy of a project?
- Does the problem summary place the specific problem in the context of the larger world? Does it describe the problem as important and interesting?
- Does the problem statement set the stage for a reasonable project to follow?

Common Challenges With Problem Statements

After fine-tuning your problem statement, it should clearly and concisely identify the clinical problem your project will address, as well as its context. Review your problem statement and make sure it avoids the following common mistakes:

- The problem is not clearly stated or is vague and lost in discussion of broad, general issues.
- Components that contribute to the problem are not well identified or addressed.
- Limited or weak data are presented to support the problem importance (and not logically organized).
- There is limited interest or need for study of the suggested problem.
- The problem is not framed in an adequate context (Leedy & Omrod, 2013).

Peer Review of Problem Statements

Again, recall the value of peer/mentor review. Discussing the problem statement (and other project components) with others can help you improve your work. As you review the following problem statements, determine whether the problem statement is well focused. You want it to be specific enough to provide direction for your project. If you were completing a peer review for a colleague, do the following two problem-statement summaries provide beginning project direction? What details would you recommend adding to either statement?

- Standardized electronic health record (EHR) documentation helps meet clinical, legal, and payment requirements. EHRs improve communication and efficiency in gaining patient information and documenting patient encounters. In reviewing the literature, no studies were found specific to staff challenges and attitudes toward EHR documentation. A problem exists in helping staff best accept and prepare to use EHRs.
- College students are a unique population. College is an important transition time, and the health behaviors students choose in college often set the stage for lifetime health behaviors. A problem exists in helping students gain motivation and action toward improved health behaviors.

Note that both statements could be improved with more specific supporting data such as literature and report references that help make the case. Further context could be added to help identify the project needs locally as well. Further clarification of terms, such as what is meant by *health behaviors* would also be indicated.

Using the Title to Help Convey the Project

The project title is the most-read component of the project. Clearly naming both the problem and the project title can promote project clarity. Again, this includes naming what the problem is and what it is not. For example, if you are naming a problem related to staff development for older adult care, there is a lot of variation with the following, "helping the frail elderly" versus "promoting wellness for older adults." These terms provide two very different pathways. Both can be of value, but early decisions as to the project's direction will better guide the project work. The correct name contributes to or sets the path for a good project.

Incorporating the problem into the project title is only one component of a well-chosen title. When your project purpose and methods take shape, they will influence the title as well. As your problem statement progresses and you move into the purpose-statement phase, you will begin to think about the overarching title of your project and how to incorporate project approaches. Being able to state clearly in your title what you are doing can help you state with your intent. Don't over-state what your proposed project can accomplish. Peer review could include asking others what they think your title conveys.

Project Triangle

It is not too early to start getting points of the project triangle to align. After the problem is clearly named and described, use of the project triangle begins. The problem statement will then lead to developing your project purpose. This will be important as you develop your outcomes and methods. For example, in a project intended to learn about staff issues with a new EHR system, a very simple project triangle might include: Purpose = understand staff concerns and satisfaction with the new EHR system; Methods = staff complete survey on concerns and satisfaction questions; Outcome = evidence for any needed staff development is gained. For reference, a copy of this triangle is found at the end of this chapter (Appendix 3.1) as well as Appendix A, at the end of the book.

Also learn from the experience of doctor of nursing practice (DNP) students who have preceded you in the proposal-writing process. Their advice is presented in the following box.

• • •

ADVICE FROM DNP STUDENTS

Problem Selection
Narrow your topic as much as is reasonably possible
- The most difficult/challenging aspect was to narrow my topic.
- Deciding on what aspect to focus on for my project was a challenge. There were so many different ways I could have gone.

Find a project idea you enjoy
- I really enjoy my topic and so the time just flies by as I am trying to figure things out.

SUMMARY

Clinical problems with relevance for advanced clinical projects abound. The problem statement sets the stage or describes the status of a current situation that needs to be addressed. It serves as the background for project purpose statements. It helps if the problem statement emerges from strong personal interests and promotes academic and career interests. This chapter suggests direction in identifying important problems and focusing them for further study.

WEBSITES FOR FURTHER REVIEW

Supporting the need for addressing your clinical problem and placing your problem in context can include relating it to data from national reports. For example, you may find it useful to relate your problem to changing demographics. Although the following reports are specific to issues of older adults and health disparities, similar reports can be found to describe other populations and issues. What surprised you as you review these reports? What ideas do you gain for helping document related clinical problems?

- *Profile of Older Americans, Administration on Aging* (2016):
  www.giaging.org/documents/A_Profile_of_Older_Americans__2016.pdf
- *Retooling for an Aging America: Building the Health Care Workforce* (2008):
  www.nationalacademies.org/hmd/reports/2008/retooling-for-an
  -aging-america-building-the-health-care-workforce.aspx
- *A Framework for Educating Health Professionals to Address the Social Determinants of Health* (2016):
  www.nap.edu/catalog/21923/a-framework-for-educating-health
  -professionals-to-address-the-socialdeterminants-of-health

NEXT CHAPTER UP

The goal of clinical projects is to improve practice. You now have a problem statement clearly crafted and, with this problem statement in hand, you are ready to delve more deeply into a project plan. The next chapter provides background on quality improvement and how it can help inform your next project decisions.

LEARNING ACTIVITIES

Your Story Related to Your Topic of Interest

One way to begin developing a problem of interest is to write about it from a personal perspective. What is your story related to your topic of interest? Why is it important to you? What do you hope to accomplish? As you identify a problem of concern, write a few paragraphs about what it means to you and why it is important to you. This reflection can help focus the problem and provide an opportunity for you and faculty to communicate. For a specific problem that you have in mind:

- What makes this problem important?
- Why does it matter? Are there important patient concerns? Staff concerns?
- What potential contributions could be made from further studying or developing this project?
- What surrounding clinical issues seem to work well with this problem?
- What clinical issues could work better?

Further Reflective-Writing Prompts

- I am choosing this topic because . . .
- It is important I do this project because . . .
- Challenges in taking on this topic include . . .
- Early findings from the literature review suggest. . . .

To-Do List

- Find three key articles that most help you make your case and move your project forward for the problem you think you would like to pursue.
- Identify and confirm a specific topic of concern that can be addressed by the clinical project.
- Write an introduction that presents the importance of your clinical problem and what is known about it. End the initial section of your proposal with a clear, one- to two-sentence problem statement that clarifies what the problem is and why it is important.

Readiness to Move On . . .

- Have you started a literature review related to your problem?
- Have you tried to think about the problem from all sides and perspectives?

- Have you considered the pros and cons for addressing this pr
- Have you gained expert advice on strategies and challenges
  planned approach to the problem?

* Maintaining mental health amid
a pandemic: A quality improvement project

* Mental Health needs during the
pandemic: A QI project

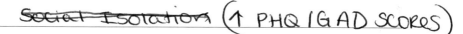

~~Social Isolation~~ (↑ PHQ/GAD scores)
* Decreasing depression & anxiety
Symptoms Amid a pandemic: A QI project

* Coping with stress
~~Global~~ Prevalence of depression
and anxiety Symptoms in adults
during the pandemic

REFERENCES

Coley, S., & Scheinberg, C. (2007). *Proposal writing: Effective grantsmanship.* New York, NY: Sage.

Krathwohl, D., & Smith, N. (2005). *How to prepare a dissertation proposal: Suggestions for students in education and the social and behavioral sciences.* Syracuse, NY: Syracuse University Press.

Leedy, P., & Omrod, J. (2013). *Practical research: Planning and design* (10th ed.). Boston, MA: Pearson.

Standards for Quality Improvement Reporting Excellence. (2015). *Revised standards for quality improvement reporting excellence, SQUIRE 2.0.* Retrieved from http://www .squire-statement.org/index.cfm?fuseaction=Page.ViewPage&PageID=471

Walker, L., & Avant, K. (2011). *Strategies for theory construction in nursing* (5th ed.). Boston, MA: Prentice Hall.

PROJECT TRIANGLE MODEL

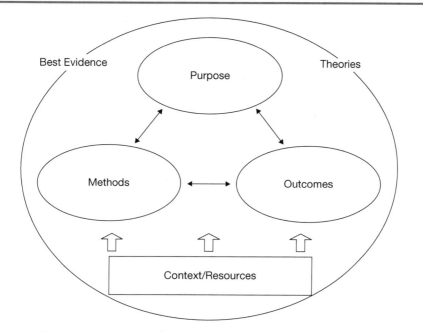

Once you have clearly identified the project problem, you are ready to use components of this model to develop your proposal.

• • •

Clinical Projects and Quality Improvement: Thinking Big Picture

Reflective Questions

In Chapter 3, you learned about ideas for thinking about and naming a clinical problem. Now the focus is on the big picture of projects, many that are influenced by the quality improvement (QI) perspective. This chapter provides background on how QI can help inform your project decisions as well as strategies to help document the need for your project on a local/practice level. The following reflective questions organize learning for this chapter. With which of the following are you most comfortable?

1. What is your perspective on the "big picture of clinical projects"? How can projects help improve practice?
2. How does understanding QI lead to potential project frames?
3. How does describing systems and populations relate to QI?
4. What are practical approaches to beginning QI data collection and analysis?

• • •

HOW CAN CLINICAL PROJECTS HELP IMPROVE PRACTICE?

The goal of clinical projects is to improve practice. Now that you have identified an important problem, this chapter summarizes big-picture approaches to help you gain focus for your clinical project. Although numerous approaches to clinical projects exit, QI is typically an underlying theme. These QI projects provide opportunity to combine scholarly evidence with a local clinical problem or issue. This chapter helps you think about potential project opportunities within the QI frame, as you begin to move from a problem area to project idea.

* * *

IS YOUR PROJECT A MATCH FOR QI?

QI models provide guidance that can improve patient care. QI has long been an important topic as it documents a type of accountability in health care, but it takes on increasing importance now with the current focus on safety and quality care needs, as documented in national error reports. Once you have identified the problem, then the focus becomes trying to fix that problem. You can ask whether a QI focus would work for you as you move into the big picture of mapping your project. For example, you might be aware of best-evidence literature indicating that preoperative patient education programs for joint replacement helps improve patient outcomes. If you feel this could be an important issue in your setting, would this be the type of QI project you would want to pursue?

From a practical perspective, QI means gaining/maintaining quality products and processes in health care, with a focus on safe/quality care for patients. QI is considered a problem-solving process that uses a model to guide its process. It has been described, as an ongoing effort to address and document outcomes to improve the health of the community. An ongoing process, it incorporates quality process and outcome indicators (American Public Health Association, 2013). QI brings useful models for considering the big picture and documenting specific agency needs as an initial component of the project planning. Points to consider:

- QI incorporates a systems perspective. It is important to understand systems, because most health care agencies follow a systems approach and as national error reports indicate, many safety concerns occur because these systems are not working as they should.
- QI involves a reflective component. You will reflect and ask questions about problems or challenges that you are seeing. As a reflective reader of other QI projects related to your problem of interest, you learn about strategies that others have tried. You reflect and ask whether a particular evidence-based protocol might work in your setting or with your population of interest.

- QI involves teams. A good QI project should be an example of good teamwork. A project might engage unit members to implement a new initiative, for example, engaging the team in implementing and evaluating a new care model or communication protocol. QI projects can help engage staff to take accountability for the big picture of care.
- QI involves feedback and ongoing monitoring. Once a project is implemented, you will want to know whether it works. Consistent with a problem-solving model, QI involves evaluation of the project and then feedback to the team. Ongoing project monitoring helps ensure needed improvements are sustained.
- A variety of continuous QI (CQI) models exist, as further noted in Chapter 7. Detailed approaches to organizing and documenting QI, such as the Standards for Quality Improvement Reporting Excellence (SQUIRE; 2015) method, are also available.

QI: SYSTEMS AND POPULATIONS PERSPECTIVES

As part of QI, understanding systems and populations provides a way to determine project needs and to describe clearly the project of interest. Many projects start at the micro-system level, for example, a pilot project to identify the project challenges/successes with a small population or on one hospital unit before extending to other or larger components of the system. When beginning a project, it is especially important to identify for oneself and others what system is to be used and who will be the population of interest.

Naming systems and populations can also help outline what you are interested in and why. For example, if you are hoping to improve diabetes care for patient populations in your practice setting, you would review the literature for best evidence. Then you might consider using that evidence to develop a checklist approach for chart audits as to team adherence to best diabetes care practices. If that review indicates a gap or lack of consistency in implementing best practices in your setting, and patient population outcomes are not reaching standards, then feedback to the team and engaging a plan for improvement is indicated. This can then lead to next steps of a QI project to help improve that care.

Thinking Systems

Systems approaches incorporate a network of interdependent components, allowing opportunity to view patterns and relationships versus individual issues (Nelson et al., 2008). Big-picture thinking provides the opportunity to identify a systems' success and challenges and to consider how these impact safe, quality care (Johnson, Miller, & Horowitz, 2008). Points to recall about systems and why they are important include:

- Systems well describe the organizations that play a central role in health care. National safety reports expound the need for improving health care systems and creating a culture of safety. Placing a specified problem in the context of a designated system helps better understand the problem and identify where specific system changes (such as new unit policies and procedures) are needed.
- Systems models, credited to Donabedian (1988), provide a reasonable framework for thinking about diverse issues with the broad concepts of structure, process, and outcomes. These concepts help characterize that organization or specific agency unit and help convey the interdependent nature of people, place, and process. Structure involves how things are organized. For example, a specific unit, such as a rehab unit, can be described in terms of its structure (staff, resources, setting). Process is the way things are done (protocols, processes for accomplishing the work of a unit) and outcomes are the products you are seeking to attain (the desired accomplishments). In an effort to understand and improve outcomes, as well as share what a project has accomplished, it is import to describe the structure and process that go with these outcomes.

Thinking Populations

Naming your population, and the individuals it consists of, is an important component of your QI project. Diverse populations are noted to include clinical populations, community populations, or other aggregates (American Association of Colleges of Nursing [AACN], 2006). Populations incorporate diverse considerations, including health dimensions, culture, socioeconomics, and environment. Documenting the population and its health is important in acute care, primary care, long-term care, and public health (Institute of Medicine [IOM], 2012). Better understanding a particular population can lead to better preparation of the clinical workforce regarding populations they will serve. Population perspectives can be important to clinical projects in diverse ways. For example:

- In a primary care setting, describing subpopulations can help identify potential issues within the larger primary care population. Knowing subpopulations issues, for example, the patient aggregate engaged with family caregiving and its related challenges, can lead to better opportunities to address these concerns. Strategies to facilitate care of this subpopulation can then emerge. For example, caregiver screening tools for individuals caring for loved ones with dementia might be implemented as a tool to identify caregiver risk for health care issues. Knowing the demographics of populations and subpopulations can then help identify not only needs for policies/procedures, but further needs in education and research.

- Comparisons of populations can also be useful in health-promotion efforts. For example, knowing characteristics of your community in terms of the extent of the risk for hypertension or stroke, and then learning that your community has higher percentages of these cardiac diagnoses compared with state and national data, leads you to ask why. You might also wonder what approaches other communities have taken to improve similar problems and review resources to gain ideas for your community. A population focus can remind one to compare data and learn from others dealing with similar situations.

* * *

PRACTICAL CONSIDERATIONS AS YOU BEGIN QI PROJECTS

Project Examples of Systems and Populations Perspectives

Systems and population concepts can lead to ideas for developing a project. Thinking of the population and systems helps consider the project's unit of interest, including its potential needs and challenges, and serves as a beginning for considering the big picture of potential future projects. Examples from large national reports can show how others have used systems and population perspectives to address select issues. For example, toolkits developed by the Agency for Healthcare Research and Quality (AHRQ), such as the Fall Prevention Toolkit and Health Literacy Toolkit, incorporate these concepts and may provide ideas for your project (see end-of-chapter activity: Planning Activity: Learning From Others). Doctor of nursing practice (DNP) project examples include:

- Wagner (Appendix C), working at a primary care clinic, found her practice was seeing many patients with chronic kidney disease (CKD) and its related risks. She was not sure that the clinic was using best evidence in guiding patient care for this subpopulation. Her project used a best-evidence checklist, developed from her literature review, to complete chart audits. She then compared her chart audit/practice findings to the current best evidence recommendations to identify practice strengths and gaps. In another example, Robinson (Appendix D), in her work at a mental health center clinic, found a large percentage of her patient population was dealing with diabetes. She proposed a QI project similar to Wagner's to better address care needs for this population.

- In a hospital setting, Curtis (Appendix E) felt that unit-based councils were a good strategy to engage staff in quality care. After these councils were put in place at a select organization, she wanted to confirm that nursing staff and managers agreed these were useful and that the system was working well with the unit-based councils. Her QI project focused on staff perspectives of the unit-based councils, effectiveness, as well as its challenges.

In each of these examples, reflections and questioning specific to a local practice concern led to ideas that could help improve quality care. The noted projects utilized systems thinking and a population focus to address their practice concerns. The projects used QI principles, including engaging staff to first better understand the problem and then generate plans to help improve specific outcomes.

QI Problem Solving and Needs Assessments

What ways will you show that there is a need for your project? QI includes problem-solving approaches that include addressing the need for a select project. Needs assessments provide data that can help describe and convey to others the baseline system and population issues. This provides a way to name and more clearly understand problems or gaps in care as well as providing baseline data for seeking improvement. Approaches to needs assessments vary, with both detailed approaches that might become a clinical project themselves, or more basic approaches that use quick available data to outline a basic need. Needs assessments help to name and document current situations in preparation for making improvements. Note that the broad literature review addresses the extent of the problem from a professional body of knowledge, whereas the local needs assessment provides the local context of the problem. Sample approaches involved in needs assessment include documenting the need as described in the literature, root-cause analyses, focused descriptive assessments, and strengths/weaknesses/opportunities/threats (SWOT) analyses.

Documenting Need From the Literature

When you first identify a clinical problem, you move to the literature hoping to find evidence-based strategies that others have used to successfully resolve a problem similar to yours. Sometimes you find syntheses of evidence or national reports that have addressed your issue and reviewed successful strategies or made recommendations for further testing. These can provide a national scholarly perspective that you can then compare with your local problem for similarities and differences.

Especially in a new problem area, one with limited study, the literature review and synthesis can be a major component of helping document need for further work in a clinical area. One leadership student wished to develop a nursing alumnae association, but found there was limited literature on this topic. She moved to a project that included systematic review of university websites and interviews with other leaders who had already developed this resource (Birk, 2015). Another graduate student was interested in developing a rural health clinic and found the literature provided limited evidence on this approach. She then moved forward to an evidence-generating project, completing interviews and learning from rural nurse practitioners experienced with these clinics (Appendix F).

Addressing the Root Cause

Analyzing the cause of events using a root-cause analysis can contribute to needs assessments, leading to better understanding of a problem or issue to be addressed. Diagramming out potential causative factors of a problem can be early steps in understanding and then resolving the problem. Flowchart-type diagrams help map a procedure or process to help identify where a process might break down. Fishbone diagrams provide graphic outlines of potential concepts or factors that contribute to a problem. These diagramming techniques can help you identify where to start or may help you rename or refocus a particular problem. A good example, which shows the fishbone diagram in action, is provided in the national action plan to reduce adverse drug reactions. Using a fishbone diagram, report authors identified where potential challenges related to the problem might be found. This included diagramming the concepts of provider, patient, and proximate factors, as well as impact of the health care system, including technical and latent factors, with potential impact on adverse drug reactions (health.gov/hcq/pdfs/ade-action-plan-508c.pdf). This diagramming then provides opportunity for further assessment and planning at the local level.

Sharing Focused Descriptive Assessments

Often applications for clinical agency designations, such as a rehabilitation specialty unit, a center for excellence, or a cancer center, require documents similar or equivalent to needs assessments. Agencies may have completed recent reports with needs assessments that help document your need and fit your intended plan. Ideas for resources and/or data for needs assessment can be gained from reviewing the noted center's designation criteria.

Community and population needs assessments are often indicated. One student, for example, completed a needs survey related to older adult community service needs to determine priorities for project need. After completing her assessment, she identified the need for an older adult transportation program; she then generated a plan to engage faith communities in a service project related to this need. Another individual completed a needs assessment of an assisted living facility in preparation for developing an onsite clinic; this description of the people, the setting, and their processes for gaining care helped outline baseline information for developing the project.

As you begin to think about the big picture of your project, confirm that you can document need for the project. To start this process, think about data that you can easily access that will help you describe a local system or a population's specific needs. Many QI tools exist to help extend the basic "who, what, how, and when," which often guides a quick assessment. Also, recall the more detailed needs assessment resources provided in textbooks from leadership or community or public health courses.

Using SWOT Tools

A SWOT analysis can be a useful component of project planning. This tool provides opportunity to better understand an issue within the context of your population and setting prior to developing a project. The four concepts—strengths, weaknesses, opportunities, and threats—provide guidance in mapping a clinical unit's issues. This approach helps to focus on a clinical unit's positives, take advantage of its strengths, and map challenges or areas needing to be improved. For example, in creating a needs assessment to prepare for a specialty unit certification, a DNP student completed a SWOT analysis. Note that in her example, completing this analysis led to projecting potential QI projects to consider (Appendix 4.1).

Checklists as QI Tools

Appropriate checklists help document quality approaches to care. Checklists take many forms and can be used in diverse ways. In general, they are intended to help minimize human factor errors and help providers have confidence in the processes they are completing. Good clinical checklists or algorithms are determined from the best evidence on a topic/procedure and require appropriate validation of design, content, and process for use (AHRQ, 2010). Although checklists are not always used as a needs assessment, they have that potential. As noted, in Wagner's proposal example (Appendix C), she used a checklist from the literature to audit practice charts and determine practice compliance or gaps in best practices specific to chronic kidney disease.

SUMMARY

QI approaches are a staple in health care; they provide a systems and population perspective. They also provide a structure and process for outlining problem approaches and monitoring quality, and remind us of the importance of documenting project needs. They provide tools for naming the big picture of clinical challenges and then framing potential projects.

WEBSITES FOR FURTHER REVIEW

Examples of resources for gaining more information about QI, and helping you gain further ideas for next steps can be found in select websites. Examples include:

- *Institute for Healthcare Improvement (IHI) open school for health professions*: www.ihi.org/IHI/Programs/IHIOpenSchool
- *Developing and implementing a QI plan*:
  - HRSA provides a five-part process in their Quality Toolbox: www.hrsa.gov/quality/toolbox
  - For those just beginning to use QI, the HRSA introductory module provides good information—Part 1: Quality Improvement (QI) and the Importance of QI: www.hrsa.gov/quality/toolbox/methodology/qualityimprovement/index.html
- *Culture of safety*. Current national initiatives provide resources to help gain ideas for further pursuing safety initiatives in your setting: www.nursingworld.org/MainMenuCategories/ThePracticeof ProfessionalNursing/2016-Culture-of-Safety
- *Standards for Quality Improvement Reporting Excellence*: In addition to detailed guidelines for outlining and reporting a QI project, project examples can be found within this site: www.squire-statement.org

NEXT CHAPTER UP

You have reviewed a variety of concepts relevant to QI projects, including thinking about your project need at the local level. Now head to the literature to determine how others have approached the problem. The focus in the following chapters includes reviewing and synthesizing the professional literature so that you can situate your project within that domain.

LEARNING ACTIVITIES

Gaining Skills: Developing Big-Picture Ideas Related to Your Topic of Interest

Consider a potential clinic, agency, or population for your clinical project. How will you address the following questions?

- How will you describe this clinic as an entity or "system"?
- What can you learn from asking the typical who, what, when, and where questions? From a more detailed assessment?
- What are the obvious strengths and challenges you note with this agency or population?
- What ideas do you have for how this system might be improved? What priorities for change would you suggest (Johnson, Miller, & Horowit, 2008)?

Planning Activity: Are Your Ideas a Fit for QI?

- What roles and responsibilities do you have related to QI and patient care? What gaps exist in your knowledge of QI? What learning needs do you still have related to QI?
- What are some examples of how you have participated in or evaluated others' QI projects? What did you learn from those experiences? What strategies might serve you in a future QI project?
- What ideas do you have for your own QI project?

Planning Activity: Learn From Others

1. *AHRQ Falls Prevention Toolkit:* The AHRQ website provides a falls toolkit (www.ahrq.gov/sites/default/files/publications/files/fallpxtoolkit .pdf) that lays out sample questions to ask as part of QI project planning. Documents such as this may direct you to components needed for your project plan. After reviewing the table of contents, select sections on the AHRQ Fall Prevention Toolkit for further review. What ideas from this large-scale project do you think might be useful to QI in your practice area?

2. *AHRQ Health Literacy Universal Precautions Toolkit:* The AHRQ website also provides a Health Literacy Universal Precautions Toolkit

(www.ahrq.gov/professionals/quality-patient-safety/quality-resources/
tools/literacy-toolkit/index.html) with an array of resources for QI
planning related to the concept of health literacy. After reviewing the
contents, select sections on this resource for further review. What ideas
from this large-scale project might be useful to QI in your area of
interest?

To-Do List/Readiness to Move On . . .

During the early preparation for your project proposal, did you think about the
following?

- Is the problem/project a good match for a QI project?
- Have you considered the systems that will be used and the population
  that will be addressed in your project?
- Do big-picture issues relate to the needs assessment and/or baseline
  data for your project?

REFERENCES

Agency for Healthcare Research and Quality. (2010). What makes a good checklist. Retrieved from https://psnet.ahrq.gov/perspectives/perspective/92/what-makes-a-good-checklist

American Association of Colleges of Nursing. (2006). The essentials of doctoral education for advanced nursing practice. Retrieved from http://www.aacn.nche.edu/dnp/pdf/essentials.pdf

American Public Health Association. (2013). Quality improvement in action. Retrieved from https://www.apha.org/~/media/files/pdf/factsheets/qualityimprovement_fact_sheet.ashx

Birk, S. (2015). *The planning of a nurse alumni association: Gaining best evidence.* Kansas City: University of Kansas DNP Project.

Donabedian, A. (1988). The quality of care: How can it be assessed? *Journal of the American Medication Association, 260*(12), 1743–1748.

Institute of Medicine. (2012). *Living well with chronic illness: A call for public health action.* Washington, DC: National Academies Press.

Johnson, J., Miller, S., & Horowitz, S. (2008). *Systems-based practice: Improving the safety and quality of patient care by recognizing and improving the systems in which we work.* Washington, DC: Agency for Healthcare Research and Quality.

Nelson, E., Godfrey, M. M., Batalden, P. B., Berry, S. A., Bothe, A. E., Jr., McKinley, K. E., . . . Nolan, T. W. (2008). Clinical microsystems, part 1. The building blocks of health systems. *Joint Commission on Accreditation of Healthcare Organizations, 34*(7), 367–378.

Standards for Quality Improvement Reporting Excellence. (2015). *Revised standards for quality improvement reporting excellence, SQUIRE 2.0.* Retrieved from http://www.squire-statement.org/index.cfm?fuseaction=Page.ViewPage&PageID=471

APPENDIX 4.1

SWOT EXAMPLE: NEEDS ASSESSMENT AS PART OF A PROJECT PLAN FOR SPECIALTY-UNIT CERTIFICATION

Brigid Weyhofen

* * *

PURPOSE

Preparing for a clinical unit–excellence application (becoming certified). Three key areas addressed: (a) compliance with national standards; (b) evidence-based clinical practice guidelines; and (c) performance measures (comprehensive care for joint replacement [CJR] patients, bundled payments for joint replacements, provider responsible for patient 90 days postoperatively). The certification for joint excellence application focuses on documenting quality care, continuous improvement outcomes, and good stewardship of resources.

* * *

CLINICAL UNIT CURRENT STATUS

Strengths: Established joint replacement program; engaged nursing leadership; attending physician with interest in improving outcome. Hospital has a unit that has been designated for joint replacement patients. Academic medical setting.

Weaknesses: Lack of training/education for nursing staff; limited means for collection of data; lack of planning surgery schedule with bed placement; complex surgery schedule with delayed cases; limited physical therapy resources; payor source limits home resources; need for improved communication; inconsistent preoperative education.

Opportunities: Increase market share; decrease percentage of joint replacement readmissions; increase nurse retention; decrease in length of stay; increase preoperative education for patients.

Threats: Reimbursement changes; ongoing financial support need; competing priorities in organization.

• • •

INITIAL AND ONGOING STRATEGIES FOR THIS "PREPARATION" JOURNEY

Engaging Key Stakeholders in: Relationship building; planning/goal setting; improved communication; partnering; stakeholder education; joint unit-excellence requirements.
Education for staff: Identification of key staff members; workday to develop care pathway; development of basic "joint" class for all.

• • •

SAMPLE PROCESS IMPROVEMENT PROJECTS EVOLVING FROM THIS SWOT

From this preliminary work and needs/SWOT analysis, sample process improvement projects emerged. Examples include:

- Process Improvement: Improved time from postanesthesia care unit to floor
- Process Improvement: Improved preoperative education for patients
- Process Improvement: Patient's perception of readiness for discharge

Into the Literature: Gaining Best Evidence and Relevant Literature

Reflective Questions

In Chapter 3 you learned about writing a good clinical problem. Now your focus is on finding the best evidence about that problem, so that you can establish what is already known about it and what still needs to be determined. The following reflective questions organize learning for this chapter. With which of the following are you the most comfortable?

- What makes a good systematic literature review?
- What does the concept of *information literacy* mean to you and why is this relevant to your project proposal?
- What are the best strategies for completing a systematic literature review?
- What evidence makes the best evidence?
- What does it mean to complete a reference matrix?

. . .

WHAT MAKES A GOOD LITERATURE REVIEW?

A good literature review is one that is systematically documented, synthesized, and situated in the context of the professional literature. Your literature review can help you narrow your practice concern in order to best name the problem you are studying. The literature also provides ideas about how much your problem area has been studied. Coping with the vast quantities of literature available involves more than an informal literature review. The review for your project should be systematic, covering important aspects of the topic, and be representative of the work that has been done. Also, a systematic literature review can be combined with an annotated bibliography or review matrix to help organize information. For example, if you are seeking best evidence on caring for new patients with stroke on a rehabilitation unit in a hospital or other clinical setting, what is the best evidence available about that care in the literature? Your systematic review and reference matrix will provide the basis for an evidence-based synthesis of this literature.

• • •

THE REVIEW OF LITERATURE AS THE BASIS FOR FURTHER PROPOSAL WORK

Gaining awareness of existing knowledge regarding practice is critical to a good clinical project proposal, and this requires systematic approaches to the literature review. The formal systematic literature review, as previously noted, should be reviewed simultaneously with the development of your problem and purpose statements. A systematic review of the literature during these two steps helps to narrow the problem, refine the purpose statement, gain project direction, and establish the need for the project.

As you write your problem statement, the review of literature familiarizes you with the best evidence that currently exists specific to your chosen problem. The literature review also helps describe the context for the specified problem and patient population. It should also remain ongoing so that the references you describe in your project truly reflect the rapidly changing evidence for your specified subject. This implies that the literature should be consistently updated throughout the duration of the clinical project.

A thorough review of the literature also establishes you as an expert in the area and enables you to demonstrate your command of the literature, best evidence, and gaps in knowledge related to your topic and its context. This means you know who are the key authors writing in your topic area, you know the existing knowledge base on the topic, and you are able to identify the strengths and weaknesses of the evidence related to your clinical problem.

Finally, gaining and synthesizing the evidence are part of the scholarship of advanced clinical practice. Your contribution to clinical scholarship is best accomplished if situated within past and present knowledge in the area. Identifying gaps in the topic can help make the case for your additional project work. Box 5.1 provides a summary of additional ways the literature will be useful in your project proposal.

Multiple Approaches for Using the Literature in Your Proposal

Although much of this chapter addresses literature review as part of the detailed critique of literature on your specific topic, the literature also supports other sections of the proposal. Examples follow:

Section 1: Problem Statement and Introduction

As you introduce and make the case for the importance of the clinical problem you want to address, this includes describing the background of the problem and documenting its significance. The literature and other best evidence can be used to help describe both local and broad contexts for the problem. As you note local issues, describe the nature and severity of the specific local problem or system dysfunction to be addressed and relate this to broad national or global issues related to the problem.

Section 2: Literature Review and Critique

This section includes a focus on the systematic literature review you are completing. Describe your literature-review methods, including at minimum databases searched, years searched, and inclusion/exclusion criteria. Also, as described in Chapter 6, you will be synthesizing your findings. This will include organizing and summarizing your literature review, often by themes; then summarizing the strengths and weaknesses of the literature related to your problem of interest.

Section 3: Your Project Methods

In this section you will talk specifically about the literature you have reviewed regarding the methods your project will use. As you critique other studies, you can gain ideas for your own project methods.

Further Literature Use in Your Completed Project

Once your project is completed, you will also return to the literature and place your project findings in the context of the literature. This includes identifying similarities and differences in findings related to your project and others reported in the literature.

• • •

BEGINNING THE LITERATURE REVIEW

A good literature review begins with the concept of information literacy. *Information literacy* refers to a group of abilities that enable you to discover information, understand how that information was produced, and use it in creating new knowledge and/or applications (American Library Association, 2016). In a practical sense, it is a critical thinking activity the involves knowing when information is needed, identifying the type of information needed, accessing needed information, critically evaluating the information, using the information for a specific purpose, and evaluating the outcomes of the information use (Cheeseman, 2013). Simply stated, information literacy means you need to locate, read, analyze, and organize the current state of the evidence or science (Galvan, 2013). For example, in better understanding eating issues experienced by patients with Parkinson's disease, you will have a responsibility to locate and critique relevant literature as well as a responsibility to report a synthesis of this information so that it is useful to others.

Today's technologically oriented world both eases and complicates this process because of the quantity of available information and the rapidly changing nature of that information. Although advanced technologies have made searches much easier to conduct than during pretechnology days, those same technologies have made searching much more complex because of increased options and the sheer volume of information available.

Although informal reviews have their place, the scholarly, advanced clinical project requires a formal review. You cannot claim you conducted a thorough review of the literature without providing the details of your search so that others can evaluate your thoroughness. Therefore, the care with which you conduct the literature review takes on greater meaning and must be clearly documented. The quality of your review serves as the foundation for your advanced clinical project; if you miss relevant literature, you may repeat work that has already been completed or fail to establish a legitimate case for the significance of your project.

Although it is easy to find information in today's world, it is more challenging to find good information. The review must yield information that can legitimately serve as the basis for your project and withstand scrutiny from the scientific community. Use of a hierarchy of evidence (Polit & Beck, 2012) enables you to identify the strengths/weaknesses of information, and thereby establish its credibility, or lack thereof. Part of being scholarly is addressing the quality of the information you are using so that you address the credibility of your sources.

• • •

FORMAL REVIEWS OF THE LITERATURE: THE PROCESS OVERVIEW

The goal of a formal review of the literature is to search and obtain evidence, review and critique the evidence, and generate an evidence summary. These components support generation of a synthesis or state-of-the-science summary of your findings as well as a decision trail documenting the process. This chapter discusses obtaining and critiquing the literature. Synthesizing the literature will be addressed in the next chapter.

The first step in the literature review is to gather relevant information with a broad general search of the literature. As you progress in naming and refining your clinical problem, your advanced clinical project will become more focused, as will your continued review of the literature. It is vitally important to recognize the review of literature as an ongoing process, rather than a discrete step that is conducted and marked off your to-do list, because as your project progresses you will learn of additional concepts and have more precise information to search. Also, the literature can change rapidly, and you must always be working with the most up-to-date information and current context possible.

• • •

THE LITERATURE SEARCH: OBTAINING EVIDENCE

There is an art to searching for and obtaining appropriate literature, and this process involves multiple phases. In early phases of the literature review, the goal is to fine-tune your problem statement. As previously discussed, the problem statement provides a succinct statement of the issue or topic of interest and provides the information needed to further refine your literature search. Early in the process you will have to make important decisions regarding the search. These decisions relate to databases, key words, inclusion/exclusion criteria, and practical/methodological screens.

Databases

An initial decision will be which databases to search. In early search phases, go beyond the nursing literature to identify how other disciplines are using your topic-of-interest concepts. At minimum, begin the search using PubMed, CINAHL, ERIC, and Google Scholar. Keep track of the "search terms" you use as you search the literature. Consider whether you need to supplement your electronic database search with additional strategies, such as reviews of professional journal tables of contents or reviews of the reference lists on previously found articles, to address your project purpose. This is especially useful in early stages to identify how others are naming and framing selected problems. Also, keep a decision trail outlining your process, as further discussed in the following.

Key Words

In addition to determining the databases to search, key words you will enter into the database to search need to be determined. This determination begins by listing the key words that come to mind related to the concept; also consider the key words used in relevant articles to help establish the initial boundaries of your topic. Another consideration is which search terms are preprogramed into the specific databases you are using as a means of organizing content in that particular system. Finally, be sure to use the search engine's ability to combine searches. Combining a search for the words "ethics" and "decisions" with the word "or" will broaden the search to articles only about ethics and articles only about decisions; combining those two words with "and" will limit the search to only those articles that pertain to both ethics and decisions.

Inclusion/Exclusion Criteria

Next comes adding further structure to your review. How will you further structure your search if your search provides excessive or irrelevant resources? One benefit of problem statements and purpose statements is that they help identify and clarify the project's scope and limits. For example, if you are reviewing best evidence on pain-management protocols, you will likely need to clarify what patient groups this includes. As chronic pain management with dementia patients has a different context than pain management for those with acute back pain injuries, noting the inclusion and exclusion criteria for the search is necessary. *Inclusion criteria* indicate what will be included in the search, and *exclusion criteria* refer to what will be excluded. These concepts are similar to "practical screens," which will be further discussed in the next section. Note that in initial stages of the review it may be useful to consider the similarities and differences in how related topics are covered.

Practical/Methodological Screens

Both practical and methodological screens help frame the topic. *Practical screen* refers to naming the types of references to be included. These practical-screen criteria could include, for example, the disciplines' databases to be considered, publication years to include, and language options (most often limited to English-language articles only). Identifying terms that you will be studying, as well as those terms you are not studying, helps avoid comparing apples to oranges. *Methodological screens* refer to those that clarify the level of study or quality of evidence you are seeking. For example, your review might note that only articles that are based on data will be included. Fink (2010) provides further background reading and direction in using practical and methodological screens, as well as article critiques.

If you are new to the process, a successful literature search will be facilitated by working with a more experienced searcher, such as a librarian and/or a content expert. The best searches are conducted by people who know both the mechanics of literature searches and the content area. Also learn from the experience of doctor of nursing practice (DNP) students who have preceded you in this process. Their advice is presented in the following box.

• • •

ADVICE FROM DNP STUDENTS

Literature Review

Use multiple search engines to get started
* Initially, keep going back to the literature and immerse yourself in multiple search engines. Spend time with a librarian.

Avoid getting lost in the literature
* Keep returning to your purpose statement and asking whether this literature is related (both formal and informal sources).
* Know what you are looking for and, if you get lost, go back to your purpose statement.

• • •

CHALLENGES/FACILITATORS TO GAINING THE EVIDENCE

Various challenges may arise when searching the literature. These relate to lack of literature, issues of accessing quality references, and tracking the literature obtained.

What If You Can't Find Research/Literature Evidence?

Sometimes even the most systematic search yields no results, and this may cause you to make one of two decisions. The first possibility is that no evidence currently exists, in which case your advanced clinical project will need to address this situation. The other possibility is that evidence exists but, to date, you have failed to access it. Perhaps you have not yet used the key terms or databases that will lead to the information you need. Optional approaches in this case include reaching out to databases from other disciplines, stepping back and using different or broader search terms, or seeking consultation with an expert.

Another possibility is that the evidence that exists is not found in the literature, per se. In this case, it is important to consider what other types of documents and resources could be counted as evidence. For example, national health care professional organizations often serve as clearinghouses and resources for the best evidence. Professional organization websites, such as the Alzheimer's Association or the American Diabetes Association, typically provide extensive evidence-based resources that supplement the more traditional review of the literature.

What if Accessing or Obtaining the Evidence Is Problematic?

Another potential obstacle is that, although you find reference titles that sound good, the articles are not available to you locally or, if available, do not provide a high-quality discussion or evidence on the topic. In completing a systematic review, you then have a responsibility to note these types of issues.

How Can a Decision Trail Help Track the Search?

In addition to saving your literature searches, be sure to keep a decision trail that enables you to reconstruct the decisions made during the search and the rationale that guided the search process. A decision trail is an objective accounting of the processes used in completing the search. This provides a type of accountability in the steps you have taken to ensure a comprehensive search.

For example, if your interest is in nursing ethics, how many articles did you find after searching the word "ethics"? What did you find when you then searched the combined words "nursing ethics"? Are you really more interested in ethical decision making in nursing, rather than nursing ethics in general? Is there a difference when you used "ethical decision making"? How many articles did you find for this search phrase and how many of those were relevant to your topic? Did you refine the search further and, if so, using what new key words and why? Now consider the fact that these questions are answered in a very short time period and the quantity of findings and subsequent decisions grows exponentially. As noted, you will need to determine a system by which you keep track of all this information.

This concept is additionally extended to what databases were chosen for the search and what rationale led to these decisions. A beginning strategy is to save every search you make, such that you have a record of the terms and search engines used, as well as the search results. Additional notes in the form of a decision trail will remind you at a later time why you made the decisions reflected in your searches. Again, these documents will be important as you summarize in your proposal the systematic approach you used in reviewing the literature. The basic tip is not to trust your memory; rather, document every step and decision in your process.

The following are components that should be included in summarizing the process used for your systematic review. Clearly describe each of the following in your decision trail:

- The databases that you searched
- Search terms and search strategies used; include a summary of search trail/phrases that led you to the articles reviewed
- Inclusion/exclusion criteria (i.e., specific criteria for this review such as literature time frames to consider and populations to consider)
- Practical/methodological screens considered

• • •

READING AND CRITIQUING THE EVIDENCE

Once your search is over and you've obtained articles, your activities shift from information seeking to information reading and critiquing. The "reading" term can be misleading in that it involves much more than just reading. Recall the vast amounts of information available today. This quantity of information requires methods by which to organize, store, and evaluate the merit (or lack thereof) of information obtained in an efficient manner.

To Help in Reading

Use active reading to narrow the field. First preview the article and then use questions to address further in reading (i.e., questions about studies/findings: who, what, how big/little, where/how were outcomes gained?).

As you read, consider the following approaches regarding how the article helps you:

- Identify common themes in the literature
- Clarify interesting points or irritating questions
- Organize/confirm thoughts on a topic

To Help in Evaluating the Quality of the Evidence

Step three of Melnyk and Fineout-Overholt's (2015) seven steps of evidence-based practice is to critically appraise the evidence. Rapid critical appraisal (RCA) checklists are used to determine whether a study is a "keeper" by evaluating the study's validity, reliability, and helpfulness in respect to the issue being addressed. Do not read *evaluate, appraise, critique* the evidence and think it means you can only criticize the evidence; rather, you must determine both its strengths and weaknesses and recognize both as you determine the quality of that evidence and its value in your own work. Most fundamental, the stronger the validity, reliability, and applicability to the topic you're working on, the better the quality of the evidence.

In addition to RCAs, hierarchies of evidence have been developed to help determine the quality and strength of evidence. It's important to identify which hierarchy you're using and to provide a sound rationale for that decision, and then to use that hierarchy consistently throughout your advanced clinical project. For example, Polit and Beck (2012) use a seven-level hierarchy ranging from level I (systematic review of randomized controlled trials [RCTs]) with the strongest and best evidence, to level VII (opinions of authorities and/or case reports) with the weakest evidence. Both Polit and Beck (2012) and Melnyk and Fineout-Overholt (2015) suggest that selecting the best hierarchy to use depends on the clinical question being asked.

Although RCAs and hierarchies vary, the fundamentals of their appraisal systems are consistent in that studies with the strongest reliability and validity produce the strongest evidence. Other resources are available to determine the quality of other data sources you might encounter in your search. For example, if you have found practice guidelines as part of your evidence search, then you might consider evaluating the guidelines according to the Appraisal of Guidelines for Research and Evaluations II (AGREE; www.agreetrust .org/wp-content/uploads/2013/06/AGREE_II_Users_Manual_and_23-item_ Instrument_ENGLISH.pdf). AGREE serves the purpose of both providing a mechanism for evaluating the quality of existing guidelines, as well as a method for developing strong guidelines.

If your search yields a systematic review or meta-analysis, then you should determine whether it meets the Preferred Reporting Items for Systematic

Reviews and Meta-Analyses (PRISMA; www.prisma-statement.org) criteria. PRISMA identifies a minimum set of items that need to be addressed to ensure complete reporting of these types of research activities. As with AGREE, PRISMA provides not only a mechanism for evaluating the quality of evidence found, but, in case the rest of your project takes this direction, guidelines for developing and reporting quality work as well.

The basic premise to remember is that "reading" does not mean just reading; it also means evaluating and critiquing the quality of what you are reading. Keep in mind that there are a variety of tools, such as RCAs, hierarchies, AGREE, and PRISMA, to help you evaluate the quality of the evidence you find. Also, remember that as you conduct this process on each individual piece of evidence you collect, you will also need to appraise the quality of the evidence as a whole as well.

● ● ●

THE EVIDENCE SUMMARY: ORGANIZING THE LITERATURE REVIEW

As evidence is identified, obtained, read, and critiqued, you will need a mechanism by which to organize all of your information. There are a number of options, and you will likely need to use more than one of them.

Archiving and Cataloging

You will need an organized and competent system for keeping track of the evidence you find. At the very least this should consist of an electronic system, either a commercial application (EndNote, OneNote) or developing your own system using a program such as Excel. These resources provide the opportunity to easily record the references you find and highlight details of the content therein.

Reference Matrix

The more robust approach to organizing evidence is to use the reference matrix or bibliography table. The matrix or bibliography table helps you to organize, gain an overview, and then be able to summarize in rapid fashion what you have gained (Galvan, 2013). This matrix or table serves several purposes. First, it helps to organize the growing number of individual articles and evidence you find on your advanced clinical project topic. Second, it provides a beginning synthesis of the literature as a whole, which will be your next step in the process. The matrix also provides the context for how your project can help extend the knowledge/literature on this topic. Paragraphs summarizing and synthesizing the findings that emerge from your matrix are then easily organized into your project proposal. The matrix itself may become an appendix in your proposal. Finally, the matrix serves as a quick snapshot summary of the evidence gathered and an easy communication tool for your team members.

Reference Matrix Format

The matrix is generally created in a table format with a row for each piece of evidence and various columns for different information about each piece of evidence. All matrices will include standard information, such as the full article citation, but the remaining columns will be guided by the needs of your particular advanced clinical project. You may include, for example, the level of evidence in one column, the methods used in another, and then place the population, the setting, strengths, and weaknesses each in a column of their own. Although you are free to create your own headings for columns in your matrix/table, you will have to include key components. For example, columns or components for the table that are often important to your project include key terms/concepts, definitions, research study methods, critique of the study, and summary of study findings. At minimum, a summary table listing strengths and weaknesses of each article is needed in your archiving/cataloguing system. Box 5.2 provides an example of headings for a literature matrix.

BOX 5.2

			Sample Matrix Headings		
Citation	Participants/ Setting	Purpose, Background	Methods/ Design and Limitations— Hierarchical Level	Findings/ Summary Strengths/ Weakness	Applicability to Own Research or Project

The matrix/table can be created using various tools, but common tools include Microsoft Word and Microsoft Excel. Sometimes a strategy that begins with Excel and then copies and pastes to Word provides advantages. Although creating this matrix may appear to be an extra step at this point in your project, in the long run it will make the critique and synthesis of the literature much easier. Also, recall that the literature is constantly being updated. You will have to consider this a work in progress as you find additional resources to add.

Final Touches to the Matrix

As you finalize your matrix and prepare to write up your findings from the literature, you may ask whether this is a reasonable matrix. Guidelines to consider include addressing the following questions:

- How much literature is enough? Have you started with a broad approach to the topic and then narrowed your topic adequately to gain the detail of a specific component?
- Have you searched at least one database beyond traditional discipline literature?
- Are you getting saturation from the references you are finding (no really new ideas are emerging from articles)?
- Have you considered whether there are classic references to include (those included in everyone else's reference list that can provide some historical perspective)?

Documenting Sources

Documenting sources and the reference format you use are considered parts of written scholarly communication. The American Psychological Association (APA) format is the tool used in the nursing profession to ensure that scholarly references are provided in an accessible format. Getting a citation correct initially saves lots of problems down the road; therefore, plan to summarize article notes (in your reference matrix) in a format that can be cited.

SUMMARY

Completing a systematic literature review as part of your clinical project is a key component of clinical scholarship. In addition, part of being scholarly is addressing the quality of the information you are using, and using credible resources.

The systematic literature review and matrix provide a beginning point to discuss the credibility of resources/references.

WEBSITES FOR FURTHER REVIEW

Finding current information in relevant and trustworthy online resources can be a challenge. Try the following links for additional information and examples on hierarchies of evidence and guidelines for critiquing articles.

The following websites provide additional examples of levels or hierarchies of evidence:

- *The Cochrane Consumer Network*:
  consumers.cochrane.org/levels-evidence
- *Oxford Centre for Evidence-Based Medicine—Levels of Evidence*:
  www.cebm.net/ocebm-levels-of-evidence
- *University of Minnesota. Levels of Evidence and Grades of Recommendations*:
  hsl.lib.umn.edu/biomed/help/levels-evidence-and-grades
  -recommendations

There are also numerous guides that can be used to critique articles. Consider the following as you look for one that you find thorough and user friendly:

- *ANA. Framework for How to Read and Critique a Research Study*:
  www.nursingworld.org/research-toolkit/Framework-for-How-to
  -Read-and-Critique-a-Research-Study
- *Open Michigan, Topic 08—Article Critique*:
  open.umich.edu/documents/nursing/topic-08-article-critique
- *California State University—Long Beach offers A Guide for Critiquing Research Articles*:
  web.csulb.edu/~arezaei/ETEC551/critique-guide.htm

NEXT CHAPTER UP

Chapter 6 is about synthesizing the literature review. After completing your reference matrix, the next step is to synthesize this literature into a document that summarizes the state of the literature relevant to your problem.

This provides you an opportunity to identify strengths and gaps in the literature on your topic. Your conclusions to the literature review will help connect the problem statement to your project purpose statement.

LEARNING ACTIVITIES

To-Do List

1. Work on the decision trail for your systematic literature review. As you progress with your systematic literature review, confirm that you are on track with each of the following:
   - Search terms and strategies described, including specific databases
   - Summary of search trail/phrases that led you to include the articles reviewed
   - Inclusion/exclusion criteria noted (i.e., specific criteria for this review such as literature time frames to consider, populations to consider)
   - Practical/methodological screens considered
2. Work on your reference matrix. To organize, choose categories that help you best capture information for your synthesis. Include, for example:
   - Citation
   - Participants/setting
   - Purpose, background
   - Methods/design
   - Findings
   - Summary of strengths/weakness
   - Applicability to your own project

Reflection Paper With Project Question

Select a concept related to your project interests and generate a question to guide your literature review. For example:

- What is the evidence for using concept maps as a teaching/learning strategy for patients with diabetes?
- What are the best practices for using debriefing as part of simulations for staff development?
- What are the best practices for using group projects in online courses for staff development?

REFERENCES

American Library Association. (2016). Framework for information literacy for higher education. Retrieved from http://www.ala.org/acrl/standards/ilframework

Cheeseman, S. E. (2013). Information literacy: Foundation for evidence-based practice. *Neonatal Network, 32*(2), 127–131.

Fink, A. (2010). *Conducting research literature reviews: From the Internet to paper* (3rd ed.). Thousand Oaks, CA: Sage.

Galvan, J. (2013). *Writing literature reviews: A guide for students of the social and behavioural sciences* (5th ed.). London, UK: Routledge.

Melnyk, B. M., & Fineout-Overholt, E. (2015). *Evidence-based practice in nursing & healthcare: A guide to best practice* (3rd ed.). Philadelphia, PA: Wolters Kluwer/Lippincott Williams & Wilkins.

Polit, D., & Beck, C. T. (2012). *Nursing research generating and assessing evidence for nursing practice* (9th ed.). Baltimore, MD: Lippincott Williams & Wilkins.

Synthesizing Best Evidence and Literature Review

Reflective Questions

In Chapter 5 you learned strategies for completing a systematic literature review, including determining the quality of the information you gained. This chapter takes you through the next step of synthesizing the literature review. The following reflective questions organize learning for this chapter. With which of the following are you most comfortable?

- What does it mean to synthesize the literature? Why is this important?
- Why is the evidence/literature synthesis important to your project?
- What does it mean to identify themes from the literature review? Why is this important?

A synthesis of best evidence provides a resource for making evidence easily accessible. Rather than a stack of journal articles, the synthesis is a coherent story of what is known and not known about a particular study area. Although large national study groups convene to develop syntheses on major topics of importance, there is value in smaller scale syntheses in new study areas.

Synthesizing is a step that is additive to the literature review. Synthesis is about describing similarities and differences in articles and drawing conclusions about the literature as a whole, rather than each article individually. It provides the big picture of what research is available (and not available) and its overall quality. It incorporates the critique of studies reviewed, but it also adds integration, or synthesis, of the results. It involves identifying strengths and weaknesses of the systematic literature review. Rather than cataloging, for example, by year of article, the synthesis provides an easily accessible summary of what is known and not known from the literature.

For example, your colleague has an interest in complementary health approaches for pain management. He reviewed the literature on yoga as strategy to support pain management and was surprised at the variety of ways yoga was defined and the variety of pain-related diagnoses that yoga was used with. Even after creating his matrix of studies on yoga for pain management, he realized that more analysis and summary of the big picture of the research/evidence on the topic was required. Because of the variation in concept definitions and populations, it was important that he identify similarities and differences so that he could be sure he was comparing similar approaches or at least clarifying the differences in the types of yoga and the variability in the populations in which it was used. This was done in addition to determining the strengths of the evidence for his matrix studies.

Just as your hypothetical colleague found in the aforementioned example, even after creating your matrix of individual articles, you will need to further analyze and synthesize the big picture of the literature to better understand and convey your topic to others. You need to use the evidence to frame your chosen problem and to identify solutions/strategies that others have used. Your proposal synthesis will include a summary and analysis of findings from the literature search.

Although the introductory section of your proposal uses literature to describe your problem and related issues, the specific literature-review section addresses the more detailed systematic review of the literature. Now you take each article or piece of evidence placed in the matrix (Chapter 5) and, after comparing and contrasting that evidence, draw conclusions about the findings and the quality of those overall findings. This chapter addresses how to synthesize, or craft, the big picture of the literature review.

● ● ●

CREATING THE LITERATURE SYNTHESIS

Synthesizing the literature involves moving from a critique of individual articles to describing and commenting on findings as a whole from the literature and other evidence sources. Synthesizing is noted as additive to summaries, taking the project to the next level, and creating information sharing in a new way via the pulled-together resources (Galvan, 2013). Synthesizing involves:

- Taking separate articles and blending them into a synthesis of the topic to help you better understand the state of the evidence related to your problem

- Showing the coherent flow of evidence of the specific literature reviewed, including descriptions of the important concepts/themes and how they fit together
- Sharing a meaningful interpretation, synthesis, and report on the combined literature findings

Your synthesis will provide a description of the current body of knowledge in your clinical area. It can help make a case of the need for, or for the merits of your proposed clinical project. Presenting this synthesis in a logical way with these steps also makes the review more easily accessible to others.

Begin by Reviewing Your Reference Matrix

The matrix has helped you organize information from your literature review, and now helps with easy retrieval and flexible use of your review (Garrard, 2013). To begin the written literature synthesis, you will return to your completed reference matrix. Recall that in your matrix, you have summarized and critiqued the individual studies. Now you are describing/analyzing what you found as a whole.

Begin by reviewing and critiquing your reference matrix and making sure that it is finalized and ready for synthesis. Check to see whether the following components are complete in your matrix:

- References are appropriate and useful and come from respected publications.
- Your findings are clearly identified from research and other evidence-based sources.
- The summary of each article is relevant, clear, and accurate.
- A good critique of reported studies is provided.
- Unique or interesting points from each article are noted.

Move From Individual Article Description to Synthesis and Critique of Matrix Articles

Typically, the first draft of a project's literature review tends to be a compilation of descriptive paragraphs about each individual study reviewed. This is problematic in that the draft is missing (a) the critique of each study and (b) the synthesis of the combined study findings. For example, if your literature review is similar to the following hypothetical project, then you have not yet synthesized the literature:

- Author 1 conducted a correlational study on stress with 50 participants and found frequent comments about crisis and specific relationships to anxiety . . .
- Author 2's descriptive study looked at anxiety. She interviewed 15 participants and found that subjects related anxiety to stress . . .
- Author 3 conducted a qualitative study with 10 participants experiencing crisis and found themes of stress and anxiety . . .

If, in contrast, you have focused more on the following format, then you are on the right track to creating a literature synthesis from these three articles:

Several studies have found that there is a relationship among anxiety, stress, and crisis (Author 1, Author 2, and Author 3). Although two of the studies were qualitative in nature and used appropriately small samples, all three support the nature of the concept relationships and need for further study.

Reflect on the Matrix Findings as a Whole

Now that you have considered steps to synthesize several articles, you are ready to move forward to a larger synthesis of your full reference matrix. As noted previously, you will synthesize your matrix via summaries of content and study methods. Synthesizing the literature does not mean just recounting the references via random listing. It focuses on a summary or synthesis of the big picture of the references reviewed. When summarizing and synthesizing your big-picture review of the literature, additional questions and phrases that may help you synthesize your literature review (i.e., as you look for strengths, weaknesses, or gaps in current evidence) will include the following:

- What summary statements can you make about the level of evidence from the various studies/reports and the findings associated with them?
- How much variation was there and how was your concept defined/considered/delivered across the studies/reports?
- How much variation was there in the outcome(s) studied across the studies/reports?
- What findings are supported by more than one study/report?
- What findings are supported by just one study, but are compelling? Why are they compelling?
- What findings are inconsistent across the studies/reports?

- What findings are outright contradictory across the studies/reports?
- What further questions do you still think need to be addressed (Fink, 2010; Garrard, 2013)?

• • •

ORGANIZE THE SYNTHESIS

Organize the Synthesis Summary Statements

Approaches to organizing and synthesizing the literature review include grouping the important concepts/themes found in your review and identifying variations in concept definitions or populations found in the literature and variations in the different studies' quality. These findings from the literature then have the potential to be used as headings to help guide the reader through the literature synthesis section.

- *Important themes*: This involves identifying each of the main concepts/themes involved and then providing a descriptor or definition from the literature. If there are differences in how the term is described, note this so as to avoid comparing apples to oranges. For example, if "support group" is your topic of interest, are you reviewing online or face-to-face groups (or both)? If both, you will organize findings so that this is reflected. Then summarize the strengths of the literature and then describe gaps or areas with limited research. If additional themes emerge from your references, the approach (noted earlier) can be completed for each theme. Summarize the commonalities and the differences for studies within each theme. Add a final summary noting the overall themes and strengths/weaknesses of the literature in describing your problem of interest.
- *Variations in concept definitions or populations*: In the introductory example, the definitions of yoga and the populations using yoga were quite diverse. Multiple studies were noted using varied concept definitions and treatment definitions that could not be easily used for outcome comparisons. Organizing your synthesis by grouping varied definitions can be a useful approach. This will be an important point to convey in your synthesis summary, noting that the current literature makes comparisons and generalizations challenging.
- *Variation in methods quality*: Also consider methodological themes informing the quality of the findings as a way to organize the synthesis. For example, randomized controlled studies with large samples

provide very strong evidence compared with small descriptive studies. Critique your reference matrix and summarize what was found. Questions that you used in critiquing your matrix findings can assist with this as well.

Note that Appendix 6.1 provides an example of a literature synthesis final summary. The themes summarized are broad communication issues, barriers to effective communication, improving telephone communication in long-term care, and potential liability issues. In your full synthesis of the literature review, you will also incorporate article summaries, critiques, and citations.

• • •

PREWRITING THE SYNTHESIS

To help you get started writing your literature synthesis create a basic outline. Outlining your synthesis includes detailing the following points:

1. Write an introductory statement to the literature review reminding the reader of the review's purpose and explaining the significance of the concepts to be described.
2. Provide evidence of a current, comprehensive, and synthesized literature review that includes a clear description of literature-review methods.
3. Once key themes or categories are identified, then outline these with specific references. Some find it helpful to begin write-ups with a PowerPoint summary. The small space for bullets in each of the PowerPoint slides force an economy of words and a focus on what is most important in the synthesis.
4. Within headings of each concept or theme from your review, in a few sentences, summarize the major approach and findings of each reference/study reviewed (including appropriate citation of the resource).
5. At the end of each major concept/theme discussion, summarize the key points supported. In addition, you will include a written summary statement at the end of the full literature synthesis explaining the knowledge available on your topic as well as the gaps in the literature. You can then finish by discussing conclusions/implications from the literature that support your project approach as a logical next step.

• • •

MOVING TO THE FINISHED LITERATURE SYNTHESIS

Write the Introductory Section to the Literature Synthesis

Briefly remind the reader why this literature review is important and what its purpose is (to enhance/support your project). Include for the readers an introduction that provides a map of what will be covered in the literature review (Galvan, 2013). Also state the limits of the review or what will not be covered. For example, this review addresses only adult patients and not children. Recall your purpose for the literature synthesis. Remind the reader of what you mean by the terms and why this is an important topic.

Include the Systematic Literature-Review Methods

Begin the literature-review section with a summary of the methods used for your systematic review. This must include the primary search strategies, including at a minimum: the databases searched, key words or phrases included, and any time boundaries for the literature. To document your review methods, go back to your decision trail and list the databases and the key phrases searched.

Include Introductory Overview and Summary Statements

Recall the benefits of introductory and summary statements. A feature of this literature synthesis is to communicate to others what you have learned. Therefore, one priority is to make this section especially easy for your readers to follow. This is facilitated by beginning each section with an overview of what will be presented and then summarizing at the end of each section exactly what was presented. Although it may seem redundant to you, it helps the reader who is not so intimately familiar with your project to stay on track.

Consider Further Uses for the Literature Synthesis

Your literature synthesis is important both before and after project implementation. Although the need exists to understand the status of the literature prior to project development (as a component of the proposal) it is also important to return to the synthesis after the project is completed. As a component of the final project analysis, the synthesis provides a way to tie your work back to the professional literature. This helps show how your project results are similar or different from the findings that others have gained with similar or related projects. Your published project can then help extend what is known about the topic.

• • •

FINISHING-UP CHECKLIST FOR LITERATURE SYNTHESIS

The following points provide guidance in synthesizing the literature and will help confirm that you are on the right track in reviewing and synthesizing the literature specific to your chosen problem. Did you:

- Discuss implications of literature findings specifically related to your project purpose?
- Use headings to provide visual signals for the reader?
- Summarize at the end of each section, describing the major themes related to your problem and project purpose, and then discussing how the themes are related?
- Minimize the use of direct quotes? Excess quotes slow the reader down, so only include the very few that are most pertinent or necessary.
- Read and review for logical presentation and coherence?

• • •

RELATING THE LITERATURE SYNTHESIS TO THE CONCEPT OF "TRANSLATING" EVIDENCES

Does synthesizing the literature relate to or include translating the evidence? Many terms and models exist to describe this process of translation, including research utilization and knowledge transfer. The common approach of initially synthesizing the evidence exists across terms and models. Different approaches may be used, but important concepts in synthesis include understanding the building blocks of your evidence (ideally well-crafted studies), organizing that evidence, and then making it available for further evaluation. Challenges and strategies related to integrating knowledge from the literature into practice exist, such as making the vast amount of knowledge into an accessible format and making health professionals knowledgeable that this information exists. Varied models have been developed to assist with that translation (White, Dudley-Brown, & Terhaar, 2016).

Nurses can translate that evidence, which basically requires synthesizing the available evidence into meaningful, useful protocols and then implementing and evaluating those protocols for utility. For example, with chronic pain/

relaxation protocols, search first for strong studies with tight experimental design. Additional data (if extensive experimental data are not available) can be gleaned from descriptive data and practitioner reports. After gaining the best evidence base, organize this information into protocol format for further testing. Further testing of evidence can be done by implementing and evaluating the protocol.

This chapter has particular relevance for clinical projects that involve evidence summaries. For example, with chronic pain management, one of the top disabling medical problems, there are a variety of medication and nonmedication approaches available. A sample project purpose might relate to determining what non-drug-related approaches are useful to people with chronic pain. For example, what does the evidence say about relaxation strategies and chronic pain?

Good clinical projects include an evidence based focus indicating a synthesis of the literature. Learning strategies for synthesizing versus cataloging will serve well in future projects. Strategies for review and critique of synthesis articles, as noted in Chapter 5, such as Preferred Reporting Items for Systematic Reviews and Meta-Analyses (PRISMA) and Appraisal of Guidelines For Research and Evaluation II (AGREE), provide further guidance for review of synthesis articles.

SUMMARY

Synthesizing the literature can provide a critical analysis and summary of the existing literature in your clinical area of interest. In developing this synthesis of best evidence on your topic, you describe the current state of the evidence or science. Through identification of the strengths and weaknesses of the overall body of research and evidence in your problem area, you provide the rationale for your project. You describe the significance of your proposed clinical project proposal and how it will extend the knowledge on this topic. Your conclusions about the literature serve to frame the problem you intend to address and the approach you propose. A good synthesis allows you to move your proposal forward in creating a succinct problem statement and generating a project purpose statement.

WEBSITES FOR FURTHER REVIEW

Interprofessional Synthesis Examples

Examples of syntheses of literature and summaries of next steps can be found in many national reports. Numerous literature syntheses (and practice guidelines) can be found at the Agency for Healthcare Research and Quality. The following

URLs provide examples of syntheses on diverse topics, completed by large professional or national organizations. In addition, the National Academy of Sciences provides reports, including syntheses of the literature. For example, obesity and its complications present a large problem in health care. The following national report shows how evidence has been synthesized first on the problem and then on solutions. Potential for further syntheses would exist, for example, on teens, older adults, and other unique populations.

- *Agency for Healthcare Research and Quality (AHRQ) Reports:*
  www.ahrq.gov/research/findings/evidence-based-reports/er223
  -abstract.html
- *Accelerating Progress in Obesity Prevention: Solving the Weight of the Nation:*
  nationalacademies.org/hmd/Reports/2012/Accelerating-Progress-in
  -Obesity-Prevention.aspx

Guides for Synthesis Reviews

As noted, guides have been developed to help review the quality of systematic reviews, a large-scale type of synthesis.

- *The Preferred Reporting Items for Systematic Reviews and Meta-Analyses (PRISMA):*
  www.prisma-statement.org
- *Agree Appraisal of Guidelines For Research and Evaluation II (AGREE):*
  www.agreetrust.org/wp-content/uploads/2013/06/AGREE_II_Users_
  Manual_and_23-item_Instrument_ENGLISH.pdf

NEXT CHAPTER UP

Theories and conceptual models provide excellent tools to help organize clinical projects. Chapter 7 addresses frameworks to guide your project.

LEARNING ACTIVITIES

To-Do List

1. Critique your reference matrix. Make sure it is ready to move to synthesis format. Can you affirm you have provided each of the following?
   - Clear description of literature-review methods and project components/processes

- Evidence of current, comprehensive literature review documented via your decision trail
2. Begin the synthesis of your literature review. As you seek themes from your reference matrix, have you:
    - Considered how much variation there was in how your concept was defined/considered/delivered across the studies/reports?
    - Addressed how much variation there was in the outcome(s) studied across the studies/reports?
    - Considered what findings were supported by more than one study/report?
    - Considered findings that were inconsistent across the studies/reports?
    - Thought about findings that were unique, but compelling?
    - Considered summary statements you can make about the level of evidence from the various studies/reports and the findings associated with them?
    - Thought about further questions that you still think need to be addressed?

_____

_____

_____

_____

_____

_____

_____

_____

_____

_____

_____

_____

_____

REFERENCES

Fink, A. (2010). *Conducting research literature reviews: From the Internet to paper* (3rd ed.). Thousand Oaks, CA: Sage.

Galvan, J. (2013). *Writing literature reviews: A guide for students of the social and behavioural sciences* (5th ed.). London, UK: Routledge.

Garrard, J. (2013). *Health sciences literature review made easy: The matrix method* (4th ed.). Boston, MA: Jones & Bartlett.

White, K., Dudley-Brown, S., & Terhaar, M. (2016). *Translation of evidence into nursing and health care* (2nd ed.). New York, NY: Springer Publishing.

LONG-TERM CARE COMMUNICATION: *Summary of Literature Review Synthesis*[a]

Linda Kroeger

* * *

METHODS

A systematic literature review was conducted. Databases searched include PubMed, CINAHL, and Google Scholar. The key words are *nursing home, long-term care, communication, telephone medicine, quality improvement,* and *nurse–physician relations.* The literature review included research studies and articles from 1997 through 2011 and was limited to health care. Articles were excluded if they were not related to health care professionals or communication. References from key articles were also retrieved and reviewed. The review revealed that one group of researchers from Duke Medical Center did extensive work on this topic. Author searches were done on each member of this group. The following themes organized the literature review: overview of communication issues, barriers to effective communication, improving telephone communication in long-term care (LTC), and liability issues.

* * *

LITERATURE SYNTHESIS REVIEW SUMMARY

Many studies have been done looking specifically at telephone communication between LTC nurses and physicians. These studies addressed barriers to communication, importance of communication, and methods to improve communication. The studies also described how structured communication can improve the quality of care or how poor communication can lead to error and liability for the provider and facility. Many of these studies have addressed after-hours phone calls in the setting of Veterans Affairs nursing homes and/or physician training programs. These facilities have physicians on-site during daytime hours. The literature does not address phone calls to physicians during daytime business hours. For LTC facilities and physicians without daytime on-site coverage, multiple phone calls are disruptive to the office staff and, unless it is an emergency, the LTC nurse often waits long periods for a return of call. Many of the studies evaluated interventions aimed at improving physician skills with telephone communication. Few studies focused on interventions to improve nursing skills with telephone communication. No research looked at RN and licensed practical nurse (LPN) roles in communicating with the physician even though the LPN is rapidly becoming the primary nurse caregiver in the LTC setting. Several studies demonstrated that relatively short clinical educational programs were effective in teaching both RNs and physicians how to better communicate clinical information to other professionals.

---

[a] Note that the paragraphs in this example do not constitute a full literature synthesis, but rather a summary of a literature synthesis.

Framing the Advanced Clinical Project With Relevant Clinical Frameworks

Reflective Questions

In Chapter 6, you learned about synthesizing the best evidence found in your literature review. Now it is time to think about the big picture and what framework will tie all the aspects of your project—the existing literature you've found, the problem you've identified, the project you propose to conduct, and the findings of that project—into a cohesive and organized whole. The following reflective questions organize learning for this chapter. With which of the following are you most comfortable?

- What is a theory or conceptual framework?
- What does it mean to frame a project?
- Why is this important?
- What is an appropriate framework to use?

• • •

THE IMPORTANCE OF THEORIES AND FRAMEWORKS

Theories and frameworks serve as an organizing resource to guide clinical projects or organize plans for change. The right framework provides organization for proposal writing as well. In Chapters 5 and 6, you learned about finding evidence and synthesizing the relevant literature for your project.

That literature helped to focus your problem statement, while at the same time providing its broader context. In this chapter, you will concentrate on placing your clinical project into an appropriate and useful framework.

The need for a framework to guide projects is universal. Consider the prospect of trying to improve quality health care in the United States without any direction at all—how would you know where to start and what to do? In 2011 the U.S. Department of Health and Human Services released a framework to guide its work on the National Strategy for Quality Improvement in Health Care (now called the National Quality Strategy [NQS]). Based on the latest evidence and input from a broad range of stakeholders, the NQS identifies three aims for health care (better care, affordable care, and healthy people and communities). Further guidance is provided via six priorities, including reducing harm associated with health care, engaging people and families in their own care, promoting good communication and coordination of care, promoting effective prevention and treatments, engaging communities to promote health-related best practices, and making quality care affordable. Although still a daunting task, the NQS framework provides broad direction on how to go about improving health care.

For the purposes of this text, the terms *theory*, *conceptual framework*, *conceptual models* and *framework* are used interchangeably. That is not to deny the important historical conversation about distinctions in terminology that has transpired, but what is relevant here is that theories, frameworks, and/or conceptual models can all serve the required purpose of guiding the clinical project. A clinical project of very broad scope may benefit most from a broad, systems theory or conceptual framework, whereas a project of very limited scope would benefit from a situation-specific theory. Again the terms *theory*, *conceptual framework*, *conceptual model*, and *framework* are used interchangeably in this text to refer to the guiding framework for your clinical project.

• • •

WHAT IT MEANS TO FRAME A PROJECT: THE PROJECT TRIANGLE

Recall the project triangle, with its points identified as the project's purpose, methods, and outcomes. Drawing on the aspect of conceptual models as drawings or depictions of a theory, the triangle itself represents a framework for the clinical project, as it connects those points with three straight lines. The lines provide the boundaries for the clinical project and enclose the concepts involved, and they provide the overall consistency needed for the project. As long as the three lines remain in the shape of a triangle, the framework provides structure and holds the project together in a consistent and cohesive whole. If inconsistency or misdirection occurs within the project, then the framework becomes askew as it consists of three disjointed lines rather than the desired triangle. In this case, it's time to literally realign by pulling back and reviewing the overall triangular structure of your project before moving forward again in the proper direction.

* * *

THE PURPOSE OF FRAMEWORKS

Frameworks serve several important purposes in clinical projects, but those purposes are so fundamental that the use of frameworks is often unconscious and their role unnoticed. Whether explicit or implicit, frameworks are invariably used to guide clinical projects. For example, in the project "What Nurses Need to Know About Sleep Apnea" (Morton, 2012), the theories are not explicitly identified, but clearly both physiological and learning frameworks were used. Another project, "Applying Lean and Six Sigma to Your Dermatology Practice" (Rice & Haycraft, 2012), explicitly describes how the frameworks of Lean and Six Sigma can be used in practice. As clinical students move on to leadership roles, it's important that they not only use theoretical frameworks to guide their own work, but also guide the profession by helping other nurses consciously recognize the theoretical foundations of their practice.

Although theoretical frameworks are invariably employed, the absence of their explicit use threatens the recognition of frameworks as a necessary part of professional nursing. Students complete clinical projects as they move into leadership positions in nursing, and they assume responsibility for helping the profession recognize the dependence of their practice on theoretical frameworks. More specific purposes of theoretical frameworks as they apply to clinical projects are that they provide the necessary elements described in the text that follows.

Boundaries

Frameworks/theories are abstractions of reality and, as such, they represent real situations in nursing. The framework used to guide a clinical project should provide a foundation for the project and establish the extent of its scope. A broad theory may be appropriately chosen to guide a very wide-ranging clinical project, whereas a middle range theory might more appropriately guide a more limited topic such as quality of life or patient education. In either case, the framework establishes the boundaries of the project.

Structure and Relationships

The framework also provides structure within the established boundaries by identifying the concepts included in the project and, depending on the framework, how they are related to one another. In a patient teaching/learning project, the appropriate framework must include both patients and teaching/learning, and it may also define the relationship between teaching/learning and patients, such that the education may vary depending on the age of the patient or learning might increase with greater amounts of teaching time. Although both children and adult patients may benefit from active participation in education, adults may need recognition of past life experiences that very young children do not. The theory may also suggest that repeating content is important for both children and adults.

Concept Definitions

The concepts used within a framework are defined according to their meaning in the framework's context. Part of your work in choosing a framework involves critiquing the model's concepts and how they are defined. This is particularly important in naming your outcomes of interest and how they will be evaluated in your project. Even a single concept, such as teaching, can have different definitions with different defining characteristics, depending on who's using the term and for what purpose. For example, some frameworks may define teaching as teacher centered, whereas others define it as learner centered. Neither is necessarily right or wrong, but they are different, and whichever framework is used must fit the theoretical definition that you are using in your clinical project. Walker and Avant (2011) suggest the process of concept analysis, through which the defining characteristics as well as the antecedents and consequences of the concept you intend to investigate are clearly and methodically identified. Through this process you identify a precise theoretical definition of the concept as you want to use it in your own work.

If your project involves patient teaching, for example, it is also imperative that the instrument used to measure teaching in your clinical project addresses the concept of patient teaching consistently with your definition. This means you must not only identify the theoretical definition of patient teaching, but also the way that you will observe or measure this in your project. Will you use an established instrument that measures patient teaching (based on a conceptual definition consistent with yours) or will you observe certain behaviors that indicate the defined patient teaching has occurred? These empirical indicators

(Chinn & Kramer, 2015) will help determine how you measure your concept (in this case, patient teaching) and establish its operational definition.

Efficiency

Because the framework provides boundaries and structure, and perhaps even direction, it increases efficiency in the project. For example, the framework provides common definitions for the concepts so that confusion about terminology is eliminated. Similarly, the framework identifies the necessary concepts, so time is not wasted on extraneous concepts or variables that do not apply. If confusion sets in, return to the framework to determine whether this or that concept requires time and attention.

Organization

With the borders, structure, and direction provided, frameworks may offer several other practical benefits. The framework may provide a reasonable format for presenting the project's review of the literature, for example, or suggest a means by which to organize a questionnaire and/or provide substantive content for the questions asked.

Consistency

Although theories do provide the previously stated benefits, they also provide a means of tying those individual benefits together into a consistent, cohesive, and comprehensive whole. The framework ensures that the boundaries of the project are consistent with the concepts involved in the project, which are consistent with the literature that is reviewed and the means by which the concepts are defined, measured, and analyzed. The framework is the means to consistency among the project purpose, the methods, and the outcomes.

⁕ ⁕ ⁕

SELECTING AN APPROPRIATE FRAMEWORK

The most appropriate framework is the one that best fits your clinical project and that fit is determined by evaluating potential frameworks for a good match. In fact, critiquing potential frameworks is an essential element of selecting an appropriate theory for a project. (McEwen & Wills, 2014). Nursing has a strong tradition of dialogue about the appropriate criteria on which to critique theories (Chinn & Kramer, 2015; McEwen & Wills, 2014; Meleis, 2012; Peterson & Bredow, 2013). For the purposes of guiding clinical projects, the following are suggested criteria for evaluating the appropriateness of potential frameworks.

Scope

One criterion for choosing an appropriate framework is how broad or narrow the focus of the framework is and how well that focus fits the scope of your clinical project. If the project focuses on patient education, then a broad theory is too general and the focus of the project is lost; conversely, a framework with too narrow a focus will potentially omit vital concepts. Consider focusing on the clinical project as through a camera lens. If the wide-angle focus is too broad, the patient being taught may hardly be identifiable in the picture; conversely, if what is visible through the lens is too narrow, then the patient may be cut out of the picture altogether. The framework must provide the proper scope, such that both the patient and teacher are in the picture with enough clarity to see and study them.

Context

In addition to providing scope, the framework provides the context of the project, and that context must be consistent with the project. If the project has to do with teaching dressing changes at home, then the theory must address that residential context, as teaching a patient to do dressing changes in the hospital where supplies are abundant and time is protected is far different from doing so at home where the supply of gauze has run out and there are competing demands from work and family. So the framework must account for a context that is consistent with the project.

Logic

The framework used for the project must be logical and make sense. This does not require in-depth testing, but may be a simple matter of whether the framework makes sense in your own experience. For example, does the teaching theory suggest that the most beneficial relationship between patient and teacher is that they ignore each other? If so, the theory does not make sense.

But if the framework suggests that interaction between the patient and teacher is desirable, then it does make sense. Choose only theories that make sense and are logical.

Assumptions

Frameworks are generally based on assumptions. This is neither good nor bad, but true. So it is imperative that potential theories be evaluated for the assumptions made, and whether those assumptions are consistent with the clinical project. For example, some education theories may assume that learners are ready and want to learn, whereas others do not make that same assumption. So if the clinical project aims to address the education of newly diagnosed and resistant teenaged patients with diabetes, who are often in denial, then the educational theory that assumes the learner is ready to learn would not be appropriate.

Useful

There is no reason to consider a framework that is not useful to your work. Therefore, the theory must at least include the concepts that are inherent in the clinical project, as well as pertinent information about how those concepts are related. Consider, for example, the project of building a house. Before the actual building project begins, a picture of the house is drawn. That picture (model or framework) provides the scope of the building project, outlines the structure and its boundaries, defines the relationships among the various rooms in the house, and serves as the basis for the building project. This picture is a very useful prerequisite for the project of actually building the house and serves to keep the project on course throughout the building process. So it is with your clinical project and its framework.

Simplicity

Although vitally important, the framework itself is not the topic of the project, so it should not be complicated or demand undue time and effort to explain. Rather, the framework should be easy to understand and not detract from the time and focus spent on the project itself. Although the student should consider the preceding criteria, there are several other aspects of choosing a framework not listed because they have little practical relevance for us and therefore do not need to be given a great deal of attention. For example, choose the framework that best fits your project and do not spend time worrying about whether it is a nursing theory or one borrowed from another field. Many important theories that guide patient education arise from other fields, such as education and psychology, and their practical contributions should not be ignored just because they were not developed within the nursing profession. Similarly, do not worry if your project requires the use of multiple theories. For example, in the case of patient education, it may be important to use not only a cognitive developmental theory but also a behavioral learning theory. Similarly, do not be concerned if you find several frameworks, any of which would be useful and appropriate for your project. There may not be just one, absolutely right, framework; rather, any one of several frameworks might serve your purpose.

• • •

SAMPLE FRAMEWORKS

There are lots of theories and frameworks that could serve as potential project frameworks. That means there is likely to be at least one framework that will be helpful to your project, but the task of finding the most appropriate framework for the project might be daunting. Remember that the framework is not the focus of the project; its job is to quietly support and guide your project. If there is one obvious framework, great! If not, there may be several that would be equally good. Commonly used frameworks include (but are not limited to) quality improvement, physiology, change, teaching/learning, developmental psychology, systems, management, leadership, and social psychology. There are generally numerous options of theories/frameworks from which to choose, and a good first step is to brainstorm known theoretical frameworks that might work for this project. Also conduct a cursory review of the literature to see what other possible frameworks might fit. The objective is not to find the most complicated and obscure theoretical framework, but rather to find a fairly comprehensive list of potential frameworks for your project. Table 7.1 provides suggestions for several different project topics and potentially appropriate theories.

Although there are numerous frameworks that can be generally considered for a project, it is the match between the project and the framework that is important. If multiple potential frameworks emerge, the next step is to determine which framework is the most appropriate for the project. For example, if the project purpose is to implement a change in care delivery, then potential theories might include systems, change, quality improvement, transformational leadership, or theory of reasoned action. But, as your purpose statement is refined and becomes more focused, you will identify additional details that

TABLE 7.1	

SAMPLE PROJECT TOPICS AND THEORIES

Project Topic	Potential Theoretical Frameworks
Quality improvement	NQS PDSA Six Sigma Lean Deming
Change the care delivery system	Systems Change Quality improvement Transformational leadership Theory of reasoned action
Improve treatment of patient pain	Selye's general adaptation syndrome Gate control theory Opponent process theory Motivation–decision model
Determining the child's role in care	Psychoanalytic child development Cognitive child development Behavioral child development Social child development
Implementing a new program on smoking cessation	Health belief model Self-efficacy Motivational theories
Research utilization and evidence-based practice	Iowa Model ACE Star Model
Patient Education	Behavioral learning theories Cognitive theory Adult learning

NQS, National Quality Strategy; PDSA, Plan-Do-Study-Act cycle.

determine which theory best fits the specific purpose and scope of your project. For example, if the purpose evolves into focusing on a change in care delivery to improve patient outcomes, then a quality-improvement framework might fit best. But, if the purpose evolves into focusing on the role of the nurse in implementing system changes, then perhaps the theory that best matches that purpose will be transformational leadership.

Once you have reviewed the project topics and theories listed in Table 7.1, think about your own project topic. Identify at least three potential frameworks that might be useful in guiding your work.

If you need more ideas and examples, there are several websites that house project titles and abstracts. One such site option is at Vanderbilt University (nursing.vanderbilt.edu/dnp/scholarlyproject.php), where you'll find examples such as the following:

- Bruce (2016), who conducted a project titled "Evaluation of a Scheduled Hospital Discharge Program" that used the Institute for Healthcare Improvement's Model for Improvement as well as Kotter's Eight Steps for Leading Change as a guide.
- Elizabeth Burke's (2016) project, "Implementation of Pharmacogenetic Testing in a Community Mental Health Center," for which she used the Quality Implementation Framework as a guide.
- Davis (2016) used the Iowa Model as the framework for her project: "Measuring Adherence to Cervical Cancer Screening Guidelines: A Quality Improvement Initiative."

Another good site that identifies many clinical projects is the Doctors of Nursing Practice website (www.doctorsofnursingpractice.org/resources/dnp -scholarly-projects), which includes examples such as:

- Dulemba's (2015) project, "Comprehensive Assessment of the Needs of COPD Patients Residing in East-Central Indiana and West-Central Ohio," for which she used the vulnerable populations conceptual model (VCPM) as a guide.
- Fox (2014) used Pender's revised Health Promotion Model to guide her project, "School Based Intervention for Promotion of Fitness and Academic Performance in Third Grade Children."
- Lome (2013), who conducted the project, "Trauma Nurse Practitioner Workload Intensity Tool," used the Nursing Role Effectiveness Model as a guide.
- Tiffany-Ellis (2013) used the Stetler model to guide her project: "Atrial Fibrillation: Antiarrhythmic Drugs Versus Catheter Ablation."

Finally, try looking at Scholarworks offered through the University of Massachusetts (scholarworks.umass.edu/nursing_dnp_capstone/68). There you will find, for example:

- Miller's (2016) project, "Implementation Barriers of the PHQ-9 in Primary Care: A Quality Improvement Project," in which she used the Plan-Do-Study-Act (PDSA) cycle.

Now reflect on the list of three potential frameworks you created earlier and critique each framework for its fit with the planned purpose statement for your specific project. Keep in mind the triangle discussed at the beginning of this chapter. Which framework fits best with the three triangle points: purpose, methods, and outcomes? As the purpose and outcomes have become more focused, generally one, or maybe two frameworks begin to emerge as the best and most appropriate for guiding your project. If you still have several good choices, one useful approach is to pick the best-known theory, as it will serve to support and facilitate the project without demanding undue time or attention. The following box provides helpful advice from previous DNP students as they considered frameworks for their projects.

. . .

ADVICE FROM DNP STUDENTS

Selecting a Clinical Framework

Clearly name and describe your concepts
- Be sure to clearly name and define concepts. This is more complex than one would think.
- There is much detail and thought that goes behind what seem to be simple concepts. Enjoy the thought process. Language has to be explicit.

Figure out the importance of theory/framework
- Theory is not my strong point. Figure out the importance and the role theoretical frameworks have in your proposal.

SUMMARY

Although theories are not always recognized, they are invariably present in all clinical projects. Conscious use of appropriate theories will strengthen your own project as well as the body of scholarly work in nursing. The theoretical aspects of your project provide an overall framework that informs all three corners—purpose, methods, outcomes—of the project triangle. For example, the theory chosen (including its conceptual definitions) must match the way in which measurement instruments used to collect data in your project define the concepts. Choosing the best theoretical framework for you project will help provide important guidance as the project moves forward.

WEBSITES FOR FURTHER REVIEW

Several websites that house repositories of project titles and abstracts are mentioned in the preceding text. Additional examples of projects maybe found online at:

- *Virginia Henderson Global Nursing e-Repository:* www.nursinglibrary.org/vhl
- *Scholarship Repository at the University of San Francisco:* repository.usfca.edu/dnp

NEXT CHAPTER UP

Now that you have the purpose of your project identified, and that purpose is framed within a theory/conceptual model, you are ready to identify the outcomes for your clinical project. Outcomes are one of the three key elements of the project triangle and are extremely important as they provide the focus for your entire clinical project. The outcomes need to be based on the clinical problem you want to address and will provide the foundation for the project's purpose statement and methods.

LEARNING ACTIVITIES

To-Do List

1. Scan the literature and your past textbooks. Identify and list at least three potential theories/frameworks that could relate to your project's purpose statement.
2. Critique each of the three theories chosen, using the criteria provided in this chapter, for its potential use as a framework for your project. Pay particular attention to the concepts and how they are defined. What direction does this framework provide you?
3. Identify your choice of the most appropriate framework and justify your decision.

Reflective Prompts

Reflections and questions to guide your thinking about how to frame your project include:

1. Is the framework appropriate for this project?
2. Does the framework fit the scope and purpose of the project?
3. Does the framework provide useful guidance regarding the scope of the project?
4. Are all of the key elements of the purpose statement represented in the framework?
5. Is the framework simple in nature and easy to understand?
6. How will the clinical project benefit from using the framework?

Activity

Using guidelines from the National Strategy for Quality Improvement in Health Care (2011), which models or theories can you think of that could help you further your review of the literature or plan for an evidence-based project related to the following areas? Brainstorm with colleagues the pros and cons of select theories for each.

- Make care safer by reducing harm that results from faulty care systems.
- Ensure that each person and family is engaged as partners in care.
- Promote effective communication and coordination of care.
- Promote the most effective prevention and treatment practices for the leading causes of mortality, starting with cardiovascular disease.
- Work with communities to promote wide use of best practices to enable healthy living.
- Make quality care more affordable for individuals, families, employers, and governments by developing and spreading new health care delivery models.

REFERENCES

Chinn, P. L., & Kramer, M. K. (2015). *Knowledge development in nursing: Theory and process* (9th ed.). St. Louis, MO: Elsevier Mosby.

McEwen, M., & Wills, W. M. (2014). *Theoretical basis for nursing* (4th ed.). Philadelphia, PA: Wolters Kluwer/Lippincott Williams & Wilkins.

Meleis, A. I. (2012). *Theoretical nursing development & progress* (5th ed.). Philadelphia, PA: Wolters Kluwer/Lippincott Williams & Wilkins.

Morton, A. (2012). What nurses need to know about sleep apnea. *Nursing Made Incredibly Easy, 10*(3), 34–42.

National Strategy for Quality Improvement in Health Care. (2011). About the National Quality Strategy. Retrieved from http://www.ahrq.gov/workingfor quality/about.htm

Peterson, S. J., & Bredow, T. S. (2013). *Middle range theories: Application to nursing research* (3rd ed.). Philadelphia, PA: Wolters Kluwer/Lippincott Williams & Wilkins.

Rice, J., & Haycraft, K. (2012). Applying Lean and Six Sigma to your dermatology practice. *Journal of the Dermatology Nurses' Association, 4*(2), 136–142.

Walker, L., & Avant, K. (2011). *Strategies for theory construction in nursing* (5th ed.). Boston, MA: Prentice Hall.

Writing Your Proposal: Designing and Setting the Stage for Your Project

8

Addressing Outcomes Evaluation in the Advanced Clinical Project Proposal

Reflective Questions

In Chapter 7, you learned about reviewing and considering theories or frameworks as a component of your clinical project, and making them consistent with your project purpose. This chapter addresses outcome choices. Outcomes are one of the three key elements of the project triangle. The following reflective questions organize learning for this chapter. With which of the following are you most comfortable?

- Identifying approaches to gaining project outcomes?
- Considering benefits/challenges to seeking selected project outcomes?
- Beginning a practical plan for project outcomes?

This chapter presents an overview of outcomes, basic principles of evaluating outcomes, and other general considerations for clinical projects. Outcomes are important expected considerations in documenting quality patient care and are important in clinical projects. They can be dependent variables in research projects or staff competencies in educational projects. In the clinical setting, positive outcomes are often related to accountability and serve as indicators of success. So it is important to select reasonable outcomes for which you know you can gain reasonable data. Too often specific project outcomes are not fully considered. Outcomes evaluation, which is often an afterthought, is really such a key part of the proposal that it receives its own separate chapter in this book. This chapter focuses on the outcomes that you will be seeking as part of your choice of project methods and tools. It includes detailing the "outcomes" point on the project triangle and beginning to consider evaluation of those outcomes.

* * *

CONSIDERING PROJECT OUTCOMES/EXPECTATIONS

Outcomes evaluation is described as addressing impacts of a program or intervention and can be considered from short-, medium-, and long-term perspectives (McNamara, n.d.). Outcomes help provide the project focus and show whether a difference has been made because of the project. Diverse clinical projects include diverse outcome components, with outcomes of a new unit protocol quality-improvement project typically different from a larger staff education program evaluation.

Just as in a research study, a hypothesis identifies expected study outcomes as the dependent variable; clinical projects identify expected project outcomes of interest focused by the project purpose statement or project question. In a research project, the dependent variables are identified as the outcome variable, that is, what is being measured or observed. Clinical projects typically consider outcomes of interest rather than dependent variables. If your project involves teaching staff about a new protocol to be implemented, then seeking staff knowledge of the protocol or appropriate behavior change may be reasonable outcomes of interest. If your project involves administrative outcomes on a unit, the outcomes might include staff retention or increased patient satisfaction scores. A public health/population project might identify outcomes such as improved symptom or chronic disease management outcomes, decreased medications, or decreased falls. As suggested by these various approaches to considering outcomes of interest, the concept is used in different ways depending on the context.

As noted, outcome evaluation is a broad topic and covers many variables and perspectives. In this chapter, common considerations are addressed. In addition to the project triangle, discussion includes outcomes as part of a systems model and principles that guide good outcomes evaluation.

* * *

OUTCOMES EVALUATION AND THE PROJECT TRIANGLE

Writing a project proposal incorporates many components, with the project triangle key in helping to align these components. Part of this process is making outcome choices fit with data-collection methods. Recall the project triangle in which the purpose statement, methods, and outcomes represent the three points that need to mesh; a key feature of evaluation and outcomes is keeping these three components (purpose, methods, and outcomes) aligned with one another. For example, staff education departments want to document that their programs have a purpose that impacts staff, patients, and organizational outcomes. Evaluation choices at the end of an educational session include outcomes such as knowledge gain, behaviors like enhanced patient care/documentation, and perhaps staff perspective change. Evaluation methods then need to be identified to document these outcomes.

When talking about outcomes, parts to consider include naming the outcome and then determining how best to define and evaluate that outcome. This relates to the definition of concepts and how to operationalize or measure the concept. As you move forward with your project you will want to be very specific on outcomes chosen and how they will be evaluated or measured. For example, in a project designed to help decrease obesity in a select population, varied approaches to outcomes exist. Examples include readiness to begin weight loss, knowledge of a good diet, actual implementation of weight-loss behaviors, and actual weight loss. You will be as specific as possible in your choices of outcomes, noting, for example, whether you will evaluate self-reported weight change versus weight change on clinical exam scale records.

Conceptual definitions were identified in Chapter 7 as components of the conceptual framework. In this chapter, you begin to think about how that theoretical concept is first defined and then how it will be evaluated in your clinical project. This means you will first be naming the selected outcome concepts and then defining what they mean. For example, if you hope to influence pain outcomes, does this mean you will evaluate a physical pain measures score or a patient self-rating on a checklist?

* * *

SYSTEMS MODELS AND OUTCOMES

As evidenced by the various quality and safety reports, this is an important time in health care to address clinical outcomes and consider those outcomes as part of a systems framework. For example, as nurses you are working in very complex health care, educational, and community settings. A systems model, focusing on structure–process–outcomes, is very helpful in naming, managing, and evaluating the multiple components of such complex settings. Part of outcomes evaluation is naming what you do (i.e., identify your outcome) and describing what you do (the process) and what structure/resources you use to gain these outcomes. This means considering outcomes as part of a systems framework. Outcomes in isolation, without considering the context of structure and process, have limited value.

For example, if your project consists of seeking improved staff education outcomes, knowing the specific outcomes you are going for helps you focus the structure/process for the educational project. Seeking the right program structure and process can help address what some of the issues may be for the program's successes or failures. This is an example of the strategy of backward design. It is part of the broad systems approach to evaluation. Backward design provides the opportunity to first identify the outcomes that you are seeking and then work backward to the structure and process of the project design.

● ● ●
_____

OUTCOMES VARY BY PROJECT PURPOSE AND TARGETS

All outcomes should relate to your purpose statement, but, beyond that, there are numerous choices in how you define these. Rather than naming broad population outcomes, it makes sense to name more specific outcomes. For example, if you are interested in health-promotion outcomes, it makes sense to identify specific outcomes for your population. Health-promotion outcomes are likely quite different for an adolescent population than for older adults, so focus on those that are important to that population.

Outcomes also vary by targets and set criteria. For example, you may not want "all or nothing" targets for outcomes (if patients are frail elders with diabetes and congestive heart failure, what does "health promotion" mean for them?). What is the specific target for health promotion? Can it be defined in terms of patient function? How broad or how specific will this be? In other cases you will be considering outcomes criteria set by external agencies such as The Joint Commission (TJC), Magnet®, or other accrediting agencies. Thinking ahead about important outcomes helps focus project purpose and methods (the additional project triangle points).

● ● ●
_____

OUTCOMES EVALUATION AND PROJECT PLANNING

When considering outcomes evaluation, basic concepts can be useful in making project-planning choices. Some points to consider include those in the following paragraphs.

Naming Outcomes Serves a Purpose

Clearly identified outcomes guide you in gaining the correct data rather than a lot of extraneous data. You will have to name outcomes that are effective, efficient, practical, and feasible. It is part of addressing the "so what" of the project or what will be achieved. Avoid collecting data for its own sake. You don't want to waste time collecting large amounts of evaluation data that will just be stored in an electronic filing cabinet. You want to focus on collecting outcomes data that will be used. Tons of data can be collected and reported, but that is not useful if it does not fit into the project purpose and needed analyses. So this involves thinking ahead about who the users are, whether the data addresses issues that are important to the users, and whether the data can be presented in a clear understandable format for the users. You want data that are usable versus just collected.

Outcomes Vary by Concepts of Interest

You want to identify outcomes that are as concrete as is reasonable for your concept. Some concepts are easier to gain true measures of than others. For example, physiological measures such as blood glucose, are typically recognized as having good reliability and validity. Other measures, such as self-reported dietary intake, are typically considered less reliable. There are differences in how objectively different outcomes are measured. For example, exercise-tolerance measures are more concrete than self-reported symptoms on a patient self-survey. That does not mean there is not value to each measure, but in the proposal you will make choices and need to defend why you chose select approaches to evaluate outcomes.

Outcomes Need to Be Identified Prospectively

Why is thinking ahead about outcome issues important? As you cannot ask and answer all evaluative questions, the challenge is to choose useful outcomes data. Ask questions such as, Will gaining selected outcome data be useful? For what purposes? What tools are reasonably available to evaluate selected outcomes?

Selected Outcomes Should Consider Who Needs the Outcome Data

When planning outcomes evaluation, it is important to address the who, what, and when. Who needs what information when? And why do they care about these outcome data? For example, as a unit administrator, is there value in creating a staff development program designed to improve patient care outcomes on a documented problem area?

Outcomes Should Have Timelines for When to Evaluate

You should also consider your planned outcomes and determine relevant time factors. In some projects it will be important to consider short- versus long-term outcomes. Many clinical projects first address short-term outcomes and then use a follow-up plan to address long-term outcomes. You will also determine whether baseline data exist or need to be collected. In educational terms, you may consider formative versus summative outcomes measures or combinations. The proposal needs to document these decisions specifically.

Consideration Should Include Whether the Outcomes Will Be Reasonably Accessible

What practical data already exists? Can you gain ideas for outcomes measures from data collection or reports that are already in place? This often comes from completed needs assessments or reports generated for accreditation or other formal reports. Reviewing similar resources in your settings and determining what is easily available can be helpful steps in your planning.

Addressing the "So What" Factor for Outcomes

Many factors inform the outcomes that are identified for any given clinical project. These include, among other things, the purpose of your project, the methods of your project (both illustrated by the triangle), and what interests you. They can relate to patient outcomes, staff outcomes, or systems outcomes. As you consider potential outcomes, the "so what" question is important and can be further clarified by addressing questions such as:

- What will others do with the outcomes?
- What difference will the project make in improving health, education or health care quality, costs, and, most important, patient, family, or community outcomes?
- Is there probability that this outcome is relevant to others from a feasibility and reproducibility perspective?

• • •

BROAD OUTCOME EVALUATION PRINCIPLES

Evaluation principles are important considerations in your outcome choices. As you begin to make plans to evaluate chosen outcomes, a list of principles that can guide outcome evaluation plans/choices is described by the American

Association of Higher Education (n.d.). Although these have been framed from a student-evaluation perspective, the principles apply to staff development, and in most cases, patient evaluation as well. These have been determined to be a form of best evaluation practices. Of note, there is value in multiple-method approaches that provide a type of triangulation to evaluation. Using varied methods as well as gaining differing perspectives from those in varied positions can add to the credibility of outcomes data evaluation plans. The principles described by the American Association of Higher Education (n.d.) are paraphrased in the following. They note that outcome assessment/evaluation works best when:

- It begins with broad values statements
- It comes from integrated, multiple perspectives and is considered over time
- Purposes are clearly stated
- It addresses not only the outcomes but the processes that lead to these
- It is ongoing (as in quality improvement) rather than episodic
- Multiple team members are involved
- It involves practical issues that are important to people
- It is used for improvements as part of a larger set of change initiatives
- It meets responsibilities to the public as well as agency stakeholders

• • •

MAKING CHOICES ABOUT OUTCOMES

Related to the project triangle, start by keeping concepts broad and simple, then work toward the level of detail needed for the desired outcome. Name the outcomes you are going for, define them, and then operationalize them (similar to concept analysis, as described in Chapter 7).

Various outcome choices are available as noted, with broad examples that include costs of care, symptom control, functional status, mortality, and morbidity (Whitman, 2003). These broad outcomes can then be further detailed. More broad outcome examples follow.

For example, outcome concepts for broad patient or staff education audiences include the following. Note that you will add further detail to these outcome choices as your project proposal progresses.

- Behaviors and competencies
- Attitudes and perceptions
- Satisfaction

Sample patient outcomes include the following. Note that you are starting with the broad outcome concepts and will later detail how these will be addressed.

- Patient satisfaction
- Emotional status
- Physical status/functional status outcomes
- Psychosocial outcomes such as quality of life
- Home/family change/outcomes
- Use of services
- Costs of services

Financial and clinical unit outcomes also can be considered. Related to financial outcomes, your proposal should make a case for stakeholders, showing that you are considering costs and efficiency to demonstrate accountability. Common measures include cost savings, cost avoidance, and revenue generation. To address these issues you will need to address the project boundaries and time perspective, define cost components such as measures to be used, and address future costs and potential effects (Kleinpell, 2013).

Related to clinical unit outcome analyses, this includes making a case for stakeholders and showing unit accountability as whole. Often, outcomes criteria for clinical units and agencies can be found in external agency accreditation guidelines, as well as applications for unit certifications. As one student example for a rehabilitation unit noted: Our nursing staff are concerned about positive outcomes for patients who have strokes. Using a systems model we use an evidence-based assessment tool to monitor patient outcomes. We use the National Institute of Health Stroke Scale as a type of premeasure when a patient is first hospitalized after an acute stroke, and then again at discharge from the hospital to monitor functional levels. Also, as part of this system, all nursing staff have to demonstrate competency in using the stroke assessment at least yearly.

● ● ●

WHAT STRATEGIES CAN HELP GAIN OUTCOME DATA?

There are many approaches from which to choose when gaining data to address your outcomes. Tools, including interviews, observations, or document reviews, are typical sources of these outcome data. Outcome data from these varied data-collection methods will need to be reported as such, with strengths and limits of each noted. Future chapters address strategies, such as interview, survey, observation, and document review, as components of your outcomes evaluation plans. Although numerous variations exist in each of these approaches, they provide a good starting point for considering the ideal and real possibilities for evaluating project outcomes.

When making outcomes choices, you can also consider the value of technology. In some cases technology can make data collection easier; for example, document reviews include accessing the equivalent of patient charts from the electronic record. Technology, in some cases, builds in opportunities to compare data with a standard. In the long-term care setting, for example, the Minimum Data Set (MDS) for accessing resident outcomes includes the opportunity to evaluate your sample outcomes against recommended standards. Outcomes on the MDS scale, such as weight loss, are captured first on individual patients as part of their electronic record (and then can be evaluated against an evidence based national standard). These data are also compiled with other patient records and can then be compared, not only by individual patients, but also by facilities with comparisons at state and national levels.

● ● ●

OTHER OUTCOMES-EVALUATION CONSIDERATIONS

Challenges can exist in naming outcomes and making evaluation plans. Some outcomes will be easier to name than others. Some outcomes will be easier to document than others. Selected points include the following:

- *Whose perspective are you seeking?* Remember to consider outcomes from varied perspectives. Address who you are most interested in gaining outcomes from. For example, are you interested in the patient's perspective or that of the staff, family, administrators, or interprofessional health team members?
- *Can you show prevention?* Important outcomes, such as prevention, present their own unique challenges. For example, how will you show you are preventing adverse events and promoting safety and quality? You might include case exemplars of what might happen without an intervention or comparisons to adverse events in previous time periods. What will you do if no good measures exist for measuring your concept? Further discussion with a mentor would be appropriate at this time.

- *Challenges with ambiguous terms.* If your project involves concepts such as "increased access" for "high-risk" patients, you will need to be very clear on what these terms mean. What is the general consensus for defining the outcome of increased access? What do each of these terms mean specifically to this project? Other outcomes, such as knowledge, satisfaction, and behaviors, will present their own definition challenges. Clarity and consistency in using these terms in your proposal are needed.

SUMMARY

Naming clearly the desired practical outcomes provides another step that moves the project forward. What is hoped for? What is to be gained? Outcomes evaluation is a key component of advanced clinical projects. Positive outcomes can show clinical accountability and serve as indicators of success. Projected outcomes are a point on the project triangle aligning with the project purpose and methods.

TIPS FOR GETTING STARTED

As you proceed with your clinical project, here are some questions to ask that will help you:

- What outcomes would you like your clinical project to achieve? How can these outcomes impact your clinical setting or patient population?
- What evaluation data are you already gaining in your clinical setting? Which are most helpful in documenting outcomes? Gaining current, baseline data to see where these outcomes stand provides a good starting point for evaluation.
- Are these outcomes reasonable and realistic? Concrete and attainable?
- Will these outcomes be short term? Long term? What challenges still exist? What is still needed?
- What would you do differently in your current outcomes-evaluation plans or to extend these evaluations?

In later chapters, you will read about common project models and common tools used in developing outcomes-evaluation plans for your project proposal. These tools include both qualitative and quantitative approaches to gaining data. Versions of interviews, surveys, observations, and record reviews will be described as common tools for gathering data to document outcomes.

You will address each outcome or each project objective and determine what data will be collected and how it will be collected. What tools will be used? What will be the schedule for data collection? Future chapters address more specifics as to where should the data-collection tools come from as well as characteristics that indicate their credibility and usefulness.

WEBSITES FOR FURTHER REVIEW

Ideas for outcomes can be gained by reviewing resources at select websites such as national reports from the Academy of Sciences. The following websites, for example, focus on health outcomes. Ideas for small-scale projects might be gained from these and similar national reports. For each of the following web resources reviewed, what surprises you? What might apply to your further work?

- *Healthy People 2020: Leading Health Indicators for Healthy People 2020— Letter Report: March 15, 2011*:
  www.nationalacademies.org/hmd/Reports/2011/Leading-Health -Indicators-for-Healthy-People-2020.aspx
- *Toward Quality Measures for Population Health and the Leading Health Indicators* (2013):
  nationalacademies.org/hmd/reports/2013/toward-quality-measures -for-population-health-and-the-leading-health-indicators.aspx

NEXT CHAPTER UP

The next chapter focuses on naming a specific purpose statement for your plan. The purpose statement serves as a focus and type of contract for your project.

LEARNING ACTIVITIES

Written Reflection

Start with a one-page written reflection that addresses your project purpose. Include potential outcomes choices and identify potential evaluation concerns. Using the project triangle, begin working backward from outcomes you are seeking to identify potential methods for seeking their evaluation.

Recalling Your Experiences

Most nurses have attended and are familiar with continuing-education (CE) programs. Think of a recent program you attended and consider what outcomes were evaluated.

- Were the common approaches of knowledge gain, change in perspectives, or planned behavior change evident?
- Were there other outcomes that could have been gained to show value in the program?
- How would you name and describe those outcomes?
- What ways might you capture those outcomes? Knowledge test? Attitude survey? Planned behavior change survey? Satisfaction with the learning activity? Other?

_____

_____

_____

_____

_____

_____

_____

_____

_____

_____

_____

_____

_____

REFERENCES

American Association of Higher Education. (n.d.). 9 principles of good practice for assessing student learning. Retrieved from http://www.dartmouth.edu/~oir/assessmenteval/tools/9principles.html

Kleinpell, R. (2013). *Outcome assessment in advanced practice nursing* (3rd ed.). New York, NY: Springer Publishing.

McNamara, C. (n.d.). Basic guide to outcomes-based evaluation for nonprofit organizations with very limited resources. Retrieved from http://managementhelp.org/evaluation/outcomes-evaluation-guide.htm

Whitman, G. (2003). What patient outcome should our outcomes management team measure? *Outcomes Management, 7*(3), 94–96.

9

Guiding the Advanced Clinical Project: The Purpose of a Purpose Statement

Reflective Questions

In earlier chapters, you identified a clinical problem, and in Chapter 8 you identified an outcome that, if met, would resolve your clinical problem and improve care. In this chapter, you use your clinical problem and identified outcome to develop a purpose statement. The following reflective questions organize learning for this chapter. With which of the following are you most comfortable?

- What is a purpose statement?
- Why is a purpose statement important?
- How is a purpose statement related to the clinical problem?

WHAT IS THE PURPOSE STATEMENT?

In the previous chapter, you identified potential outcomes for your clinical project. Now you'll turn to writing the purpose statement that will address the clinical problem and provide continued direction throughout the duration of the project. For example, if the clinical problem is inconsistency in orienting patients to cardiac rehabilitation, such that vital content is sometimes missed or care is not individualized enough, then the purpose statement should direct the project by addressing that problem and finding an answer. In this case, taking the problem statement to the next level includes generating a purpose statement that guides the project toward resolving the problem with cardiac rehabilitation orientation. You may have to consider solutions or strategies for further study of that problem, and these reflections will lead your thinking and writing to a clear purpose statement for your project. For example, the purpose in this case may be to develop a template to guide development and testing of future new cardiac rehabilitation orientation exemplars.

The purpose statement provides guidance and direction throughout the project. You may propose to develop evidence-based protocols for managing chronic health problems, to develop evidence-based education programs to guide staff in gaining competencies, or to generate new evidence related to unique patient population needs. Regardless of the project proposed, there will undoubtedly be times of confusion and misdirection as you progress. It is at these times that the purpose statement is essential to redirecting focus to the proposed project. For example, lost in the volumes of literature on cardiac rehabilitation, you may find yourself reviewing evidence relating to pediatrics and wondering whether that's how you should be spending your time. Return to the purpose statement and determine whether the population identified includes pediatrics or not. If adults are specified in the purpose statement, then you need to redirect your literature review to focus on adults. If at any time there is a question about the direction in which the project is progressing, return to the purpose statement and see whether there is a match.

• • •

THE PROJECT TRIANGLE

The project triangle uses the purpose statement to ensure that the clinical problem is addressed and to keep all elements of the project consistent with one another and with the project as a whole. Recall that the three points represent the purpose statement, methods, and outcomes. As you progress through the advanced clinical project, those three points should remain intact, indicating consistency among the purpose, methods, and outcomes. Note that the purpose statement is deliberately positioned at the top of the triangle; it might even be considered analogous to the North Star in providing direction and guidance throughout the project. For example, in the project to develop and test an orientation template for new cardiac rehabilitation patients, one method may include an evidence review of the literature for orientation template development, a cardiovascular exemplar completed with peer review, and then piloting with new patients. When direction is lost or you begin to flounder, which will invariably happen, simply look to the top of the triangle and review the purpose statement. The rest of the project should be consistent with and support that purpose statement.

* * *

HOW IS A PURPOSE STATEMENT RELATED TO THE CLINICAL PROBLEM?

You identified an outcome in Chapter 8 that, if achieved, would address your clinical problem and improve the quality of patient care. The next step is to take that problem statement and outcome and translate them into a purpose statement. In the purpose statement you take an existing clinical problem statement and translate it into a statement that will guide you into a future resolution (outcome) of the problem. Thus, addressing the purpose statement will answer the clinical problem identified (Dusick, 2011) and produce the desired outcome.

Just as naming the problem and reviewing the literature occurred together, as discussed in earlier chapters, the development of the purpose statement also occurs simultaneously with the literature review. As the purpose statement represents the future answer to a current clinical problem, it is important that current information about the problem is known and accounted for in the project. It is also important that enough literature be reviewed to establish the clinical relevance and value of the proposed clinical project. When completed and reviewed, the purpose statement should confirm the focus and value of the clinical project in terms of addressing the identified problem statement and also contributing to the best current evidence in clinical practice.

* * *

PROBLEM STATEMENT TO PURPOSE STATEMENT

From Problem to Solution

You are now ready to move from a clinical problem that needs to be addressed in order to improve patient care (your problem statement) to a project purpose that will solve that problem (your purpose statement). For example, the lack of evidence supporting the use of simulation in the hospital orientation of new graduates may be the problem to solve, and generating evidence about the effectiveness of simulation experiences to guide graduate nurses in the 3-month new-hospital-employee orientation would be an appropriate way to state the purpose that would address that problem.

Although it is preferable for purpose statements to provide details of the project, it may be helpful to first practice the transition from problem statement to general-purpose statement, from problem to solution. Remember the nurse who did not have a consistent or thorough orientation for new cardiac rehabilitation patients? Think about what the solution to that problem would be in order to start writing the purpose statement. In this case, the purpose statement might be to conduct a comprehensive literature review in order to establish a new orientation protocol. Do you see the transition from a clinical problem (an inconsistent orientation for new cardiac rehabilitation patients) to a project that addresses the problem (a literature review to establish an orientation protocol)? Another example might be as follows: You are using simulation to orient new-graduate nurses to the hospital, but you are not sure whether it is an effective method of orientation. That problem might translate into the following project purpose statement: To generate evidence regarding the effectiveness of the simulation experiences for new nursing staff and to identify implications for future orientation sessions.

An Optional Approach for Getting Started: The Clinical Question

First steps can be very difficult. When moving from the clinical problem to the purpose statement, you are moving from a problem that needs to be solved to a future project that will address that problem. Sometimes a helpful step in moving from the clinical problem statement to the purpose statement is to first convert the clinical problem into a clinical question, which implies a future response and, in turn, represents your project's purpose. In addition to helping you clarify the desired outcomes of your advanced clinical project, the clinical question can also provide a reasonable starting point for a literature search. Note that the way the clinical problem is stated makes a big difference in the topic that's addressed and the answer that will be found. Melnyk and Fineout-Overholt's (2014) PICOT (population, intervention, comparison, outcomes, and time) questions provide a sample format that demonstrates this principle for reviewing the literature. Perhaps you've implemented simulations into the hospital orientation for new nurses, and the clinical problem you need to address is whether use of simulations provides an adequate orientation experience. Note the nuances in the following questions asked and the answers that will be produced.

- For graduate nurses taking a 3-month new-hospital-employee orientation program, how do clinical experiences versus simulated experiences affect skill acquisition and critical thinking skills?

- For graduate nurses taking a 3-month new-hospital-employee orientation program, do simulated experiences compared with clinical experiences lead to more accuracy diagnosing at-risk new-graduate employees?
- How do graduate nurses in a 3-month new-hospital-employee orientation program perceive simulated experiences?

Again the PICOT questions may guide your literature search and help you identify the level of literature/research evidence available relevant to the clinical problem you've identified. In fact, they may be most useful in guiding the literature review, rather than providing further project direction, because of the limited number of well-developed studies in so many diverse areas of nursing. Now reflect on the three clinical questions just posed and consider the purpose statement that might flow from each. For example, if your clinical question is about how graduate nurses perceive simulated experiences, then your purpose statement might read:

- The purpose of this project is to describe how graduate nurses perceive simulated experiences as part of their 3-month new-hospital-employee orientation program.

Keep in mind that different clinical problems and questions can lead to various purpose statements; therefore, make sure you write the purpose statement to answer the question you really want to be answered.

Revising Your Purpose Statement

Keep in mind that the first draft of your purpose statement will not be your final purpose statement. The initial leap from problem statement to general-purpose statement is a vital exercise in transitioning from current problem to future project solution. However, once that initial step is taken, there will likely be multiple iterations as you move from an initial purpose statement to a fully mature and well-expressed purpose statement.

Also, be aware that revising your initial statement into a good purpose statement is harder than it might look at first glance. Take, for example, the following statement: The purpose of this project is to develop a teaching tool for new hospital nurses. This statement leaves the reader with more questions than answers. What is the topic of the teaching tool? A teaching tool for a skills lab would be very different from a teaching tool about hospital policies. What level of new nurses? A teaching tool for new graduates would be very different from one for seasoned nurses. Once you have an initial purpose statement written, read it over several times and ask yourself what's missing. That missing information provides direction for your subsequent purpose-statement revisions. After considering the following purpose statements, identify missing information, and revise each statement to provide the missing information.

The purpose of this clinical project is to:

- Implement a new simulation scenario for practicing nurses
- Improve the quality of care for patients hospitalized in the Midwest
- Evaluate peer-led support groups for newly diagnosed teenage diabetics

The Final Purpose Statement

Although it would be nice for purpose statements to answer every who, what, when, where, and how question, sometimes that is not feasible. Minimally, the purpose statement should be honed down to a single concise statement, written explicitly as the purpose statement, which identifies the project topic and population. Preferably it will also include the methods to be used, variables involved, and the setting (Cambridge Rindge & Latin School [CRLS], 2009; Dusick, 2011). An example of a good purpose statement is as follows: "The purpose of this study is to develop an evidence-based protocol regarding the use of simulation experiences to optimize skill acquisition and critical thinking in a 3-month new-graduate nurse hospital-orientation program." Note that this purpose statement includes the topic (simulation), method (evidence based with a review of literature), the concepts (simulation, skill acquisition, and critical thinking), the population (new-graduate nurses), the setting (hospital orientation), and the outcome (skills acquisition and critical thinking). Again, reflect on the nuances of this purpose statement and the way in which subtle changes might affect the nature of the project and the outcomes obtained.

The final question to ask yourself as you revise and refine your purpose statement is: If I conduct this project, will the clinical problem I started with be addressed or resolved? Assuming skill acquisition and critical thinking are the two outcomes you're interested in, this purpose statement will produce an outcome that answers the clinical problem originally identified, so you are ready to move forward to mapping out your clinical project. But if not, stop now before investing more time in the wrong project and back up to your clinical problem. Rework the previous steps, explore the fine nuances in the clinical question you want to answer, and rewrite the purpose statement until it describes the work you need to do to resolve the clinical problem you initially identified.

• • •

CHECKLIST: EVALUATING THE PURPOSE STATEMENT

Recall that the problem statement and outcome are inextricably linked to the purpose statement. After you have written an initial purpose statement, revised it, and decided on your final version, then answer the following yes-or-no questions:

1. Are you attempting to solve the right problem? Have you looked at the issue from multiple perspectives (such as people, place, and process factors) and considered the best approach for focusing your project?
2. Is the project purpose stated completely? Does it incorporate the proposed population, any proposed intervention, and proposed outcomes?
3. Have you read enough literature relevant to your topic to know that your project purpose has relevance?
4. Is it clear how the project will be limited or focused to make it manageable?
5. Does the purpose statement have the potential for providing important and useful information to improve clinical practice?
6. Does the purpose statement lead to the desired outcome?
7. Is the purpose focused enough to be accomplished with a reasonable expenditure of time, money, and effort?
8. Have you considered potential pitfalls?
9. Will the project have the potential to advance clinical processes or outcomes in an important way?
10. Look at the purpose statement once more and ask yourself: Is this project really what I want to focus on?

If you answer each question with a resounding "yes," then you're ready to move forward. Any "no" responses indicate a need for further reflection and likely additional revisions to the purpose statement.

• • •

ADDITIONAL STEPS IN WRITING THE PURPOSE STATEMENT

There are two additional steps in writing a good purpose statement. First, continue to review your purpose statement and make appropriate revisions and repeat this activity on several different occasions. Time does make a difference, so when you believe you have your final purpose statement, come back to it at several different times to make sure it still passes the yes/no questions checklist.

Second, ask a colleague to review your purpose statement and provide feedback. Give this step serious thought, considering the strengths various colleagues have to offer in this process, and decide on those people who have the most to offer. Choose peers who will provide honest, if gentle, constructive criticism rather than those who will just provide the easier-to-give (and receive) compliments. With an initial list in hand, begin a thorough process of identifying the best candidates to recruit for this important job:

- What are the person's strengths in terms of content?
- What are the person's strengths in terms of interpersonal skills?
- What limitations does the person have in terms of time, content, and interactions?
- Will the person provide honest feedback?
- Are there other factors to consider?

This objective review will likely result in needed revisions that you would otherwise miss. Have more than one other person review the purpose statement, preferably a nurse and a nonnurse colleague, as this offers a broader review and greater variety of perspectives to provide input. Keep in mind that this step may take more time than expected depending on your reviewers' respective schedules, so build that time into your own project timeline. Also keep in mind the thoughts of previous doctor of nursing practice (DNP) students as they wrestled with their own purpose statements, as presented in the following box.

● ● ●

ADVICE FROM DNP STUDENTS

Purpose Statements

Use the purpose statement to keep your project focused
- The most important thing I learned was how to narrow the focus of my project.

Keep the purpose statement in front of you at all times
- Keep the purpose of the project in mind.
- If the beginning section of the project is not aligned (correctly focused with the purpose), then it misaligns the entire project.
- From general idea to specific problem, writing a succinct purpose statement—including the concepts in a context—becomes clear as the proposal unfolds.

SUMMARY

This chapter has provided a thorough guide in moving your problem statement to the purpose statement you will use for your proposal. Consider the significance of the purpose statement and its importance to clinical practice. Would you be enthused about working on this proposal? If it were addressed, would patient care be improved?

WEBSITES FOR FURTHER REVIEW

How others have focused purpose statements and project questions can be helpful in gaining ideas and thinking through your own project. Examples of resources for gaining further ideas about purpose statements and project questions can be found at the following URL.

- *Professional Practice—Ask a Clinical Question (Nurse Anesthetist Association)*: www.aana.com/resources2/professionalpractice/Pages/Ask-A-Clinical -Question.aspx

NEXT CHAPTER UP

You now have a clearly written purpose statement that links your project to a clinical problem and guides your project as it resolves that problem by attaining the desired outcome. The next step is to map out your clinical project, from the purpose statement to the findings, including all of the intervening activities. Remember that the methods and data-collection plans must remain consistent with the problem, outcomes, and purpose statement. Also keep in mind that, although anticipating potential problems and laying the groundwork for your final project paper takes more time now, both will prove to be the most efficient means of implementing and completing your clinical project.

LEARNING ACTIVITIES

To-Do List

1. Think back to Chapter 3 when you identified potential clinical problems and wrote problem statements. Select three of your ideas from that chapter and take the leap from the problem statement (which you

previously wrote) to an initial purpose statement. Evaluate your initial purpose statement by asking yourself the following two questions:

    a. Do you see the transition from an existing clinical problem to a project that, if conducted, would address that clinical problem?

    b. If the project were conducted, would it solve your clinical problem?

2. Go back to your three initial purpose statements and ask yourself what's missing. Is there information about the topic? Population? Methods? Concepts or variables? Setting? Outcome? Make appropriate revisions by adding in the missing information.

3. Review the three revised purpose statements and evaluate each according to the evaluation (yes/no questions) checklist. Make appropriate revisions.

4. Identify three professional peers and ask for their constructive feedback on the purpose statements.

Peer-Review Activity

Place yourself in the role of providing peer review for a colleague's advanced clinical project purpose statement. What suggestions would you make to your colleague for improving these initial purpose statements?

- Implement a new policy for breastfeeding mothers
- Establish protocols for psychiatric patients
- Improve safety with elderly patients on the orthopaedic unit
- Reduce medication errors in the extended-care facility
- Provide better care for patients with anxiety

_____

_____

_____

_____

_____

REFERENCES

Cambridge Rindge & Latin School. (2009). Writing a statement of purpose. Retrieved from http://www.crlsresearchguide.org/09_writing_state_of_purp.asp

Dusick, D. M. (2011). Bold educational software: Writing the purpose statement. Retrieved from http://bold-ed.com/barrc/problem.htm

Melnyk, B. M., & Fineout-Overholt, E. (2014). *Evidence-based practice in nursing & healthcare: A guide to best practice* (3rd ed.). Philadelphia, PA: Wolters Kluwer/ Lippincott Williams & Wilkins.

10

Mapping It Out, From Problem to
Advanced Clinical Project Plan

Reflective Questions

In Chapter 9 you created a clear purpose statement for your intended project. This chapter guides you in mapping out the big picture of your clinical project. You will be generating ideas for achieving your proposed purpose statement and laying the groundwork for the full project. The following reflective questions organize learning for this chapter. With which of the following are you most comfortable?

- What strategies for framing evidence-based projects are available?
- What is your rationale for proposing varied evidence-based projects?
- How will you begin to outline project-proposal plans?

This chapter is about beginning to design and map out your clinical project proposal. The concept of project design (methods) is key. Designing means setting the stage for the project/study. In many cases, the well-designed clinical project can be one step in a change process for improving clinical outcomes. Multiple models exist to guide evidence-based practice (Melnyk & Fineout-Overholt, 2014). This chapter describes some commonly used examples.

Clinical projects involve using the best evidence and project tools to help improve patient care. They also involve choosing from various possibilities. The primary questions that the clinical project addresses are:

1. What is the problem?
2. What is the current evidence?
3. Given the state of evidence, what will be your project focus or purpose statement?
4. What are the projected outcomes of interest? How will you evaluate what happened?
5. What type of design best helps frame the project? What project approaches will be needed?

As you address your proposal, you have already started to answer questions 1 through 4 in previous chapters. For example, as director of continuing education (CE) for the house, you know that more education on palliative care for your long-term care setting is important. After completing your systematic literature review, you found that although there was broad information/ evidence on palliative care, there was limited information on specific topics such as nutrition and eating issues at the end of life. From your work in this area you know this is an aspect of both family and staff concern. So, in summary, you have identified a problem, reviewed the current evidence in the literature, considered possible outcomes, and have written a purpose statement based on the problem and evidence.

Now, in this chapter, you will address questions regarding the state of evidence and, given that evidence, determine what methods are appropriate in structuring that project. So mapping the plan should fit the problem and status of the evidence. Evidence and theory then serve as starting points to map out your project to meet your selected goals and outcomes. In many ways, your project is focused for you by determining the level of quality evidence available. If extensive evidence exists and evidence synthesis is needed, that is one approach. If evidence-based protocols are found that can direct practice, then another approach is indicated. If limited evidence exists, consider theory-based or basic descriptive approaches for helping to further generate evidence.

Mapping out the clinical project proposal also requires you to look at the big picture or sketch out the whole. This helps you look for your best approach to an evidence-based project, as well as potential glitches in the plan that could otherwise be overlooked until it is too late to make a correction for a meaningful project. It reminds you to assess the level of evidence before determining a project type. It helps you clarify how the project will roll out.

● ● ●

MAPPING IT OUT AND WHAT THAT MEANS

From prior educational experience, recall that if you don't have a plan or map, it is much harder to find your way. It is important to map out your project proposal so that you don't get lost. In this chapter, you will be working on a big picture or map of your project. Your map helps form the big picture; further details of more specific methods are described once this map is designed.

Being prospective in mapping the project helps minimize potential problems by gaining early guidance and clarifying proposal expectations; it provides an opportunity to act in advance to deal with anticipated challenges. Although mapping out the project prospectively may seem an unnecessary use of time now, its benefit down the road will be obvious, including time saved in the long run and reduced numbers of problems encountered along the way. Again, to begin mapping, recall the state of the evidence on your topic. You will also consider broad project models, such as quality improvement, descriptive surveys, and case studies, to help choose a logical project pathway.

● ● ●

RECALLING THE STATE OF THE EVIDENCE

Before mapping your project plan, you have to consider your problem/topic and the stage at which the available evidence is currently. That will then direct the project methods and outcomes. What if a concern emerged about pain management for patients with dementia? What approaches to a project proposal would be best? Surveying staff knowledge, synthesizing the evidence, or implementing an evidence-based protocol on pain management might all be possible choices. Which one makes the best sense? If, for example, after reviewing the literature on pain-management issues for patients with late-stage dementia, you find the following:

1. Good evidence on the topic in varied articles but it is not well synthesized; then you will focus on developing an evidence synthesis or a summary protocol of available data. This will lead to a next step, such as protocol development or checklists for further testing. This is referred to as an *evidence synthesis plus* project.
2. Extensive evidence and protocols exist on the topic; you might then implement or evaluate an evidence-based protocol in your specified setting, using approaches such as quality improvement. This is often referred to as an *evidence-implementing or evaluating* project.
3. Limited articles/evidence on the topic exist; then you will conduct a project that generates evidence, for example, a project that gains

information from families/staff about the problem/concept. This is often referred to as an *evidence-generating* project.

• • •

PROJECT MAPPING: DETERMINING A PROJECT PATHWAY FOR AN EVIDENCE-BASED CLINICAL PROJECT

When writing your project proposal, it helps first to identify a big picture of your plans/methods and then focus in on a tight description of a clinical project that can be carried out step by step. The approach for your project proposal (and mapping it out) depends in large part on your literature review and what evidence is available on your topic. The three types of projects noted previously—evidence synthesizing, evidence implementing, and evidence generating—will be used to organize this section as you consider their potential in mapping your project. Appendix 10.1 provides a generic template to help you begin your work.

Why Evidence Synthesis Plus Approaches?

Synthesis of the literature involves making the best evidence easily available to health-professional staff. Especially in new areas of study, the literature synthesis can be a major component of a project. It can lead to developing products such as best-evidence checklists, protocols, or decision trees (Box 10.1).

BOX 10.1

Quick Outline: Proposing an Evidence Synthesis Plus Project

Use the following considerations to determine whether the synthesis approach to generating an evidence-based product, such as an evidence-based checklist for chart review or protocol, is reasonable for your specialty situation.

* *Current available evidence*: If you are finding quite a bit of research literature on your focused problem, and you are asking questions such as: Is my topic or problem one that has a lot of evidence in

(continued)

BOX 10.1 *(continued)*

the literature? One that is ripe for synthesis of what is known in nursing or other disciplines? One for which I can access sources of best evidence?

- *Context*: In concert with the literature, the need exists for this project in a specific population and setting. This need can be reasonably described.
- *Possible methods*: Systematic review and synthesis of the literature, including expert review of process and outcomes. You then synthesize recommendations for practice and/or identify needs for further research. The Academic Center for Evidence-Based Practice (ACE) Star Model provides a visual of moving through these components (ACE, 2013).
- *Further reading*: Chapters 5 and 6 provide an introduction to literature synthesis. Other recommendations include books and resources on synthesizing the literature, generating checklists, and protocols.
- *Evidence synthesis plus examples*: Examples might include synthesizing the literature and developing a guideline on meeting patients' end-of-life nutrition needs for long-term care nurses. Or it might include a review of the evidence specific to the needs of pediatric patients with obesity and a checklist of nursing considerations if they are having anesthesia/surgery (see proposal abstract—Appendix G). Another example includes developing a checklist of best practices in care of the patient with chronic kidney disease (see Appendix C).

These systematic reviews of the literature can help guide clinician decisions, inform patient choices, and help others (professional organizations and payers) better understand and use best clinical evidence. These evidence-synthesizing projects can address populations and systems issues and generate resources to meet their needs. These projects can serve as a step in translating research to practice. New evidence-based checklists or protocols that promote safe-care delivery and products for education and leadership are examples. A summary of an evidence synthesis plus project relevant to pediatric patients and surgical anesthesia is provided in Appendix G.

In another proposal abstract focusing on quality improvement, a student found what she thought was a problem with lack of follow-up of chronic kidney disease in her primary care setting. Her evidence synthesis plus proposal combined a literature synthesis with generation of a checklist of best practices that she was then able to use for clinic chart review to document process improvement needs (see Appendix C).

Once an evidence-synthesizing approach has been determined, synthesizing the relevant literature is the next step. Products for this type of project include a synthesis document that provides the basis for further project development such as a protocol/guide ready for further testing. These products are based on systematic reviews that include a critique of the evidence. The synthesis product is then evaluated before it is recommended as ready for practice. A number of models for developing systematic reviews and further products exist, such as the Stetler model for translating evidence. Melnyk and Fineout-Overholt (2014) describe these models and their similar phases, which include:

- Preparation (of the systematic literature review, which involves the steps: search/sort/select/evaluate and then synthesize common findings)
- Validation of the review with some type of expert or process/content review
- Translation of the review for an application product of some type
- Evaluation phase for the product implementation

Why Evidence-Implementing and Evaluating Approaches?

Perhaps in your literature review you find the evidence has already been synthesized into a protocol by a respected source. The question becomes: Does the protocol work in all settings with all specialty populations? Will it work for your setting and population? Evidence implementing and evaluating basically means testing an established evidence-based protocol. It involves asking questions such as do these protocols work in your specified setting?

These types of projects are often framed as quality-improvement projects, change projects, or they use a case study/case report approach. The quality-improvement approach, for example, would include showing the need for your identified protocol, the strategy for implementing it, and how it would be evaluated. Appendix H provides an example of testing an established staff/provider communication protocol in a unique long-term care setting. The case study or case report frame might be another consideration for organizing this type of project. Box 10.2 summarizes this approach.

BOX 10.2

Quick Outline: Proposing an Evidence-Implementing and Testing Project

- *Current available evidence*: High-quality evidence exists in the form of a protocol from a well-respected source. You might choose this approach if, after reviewing this protocol, you wonder whether it has relevance and would work on a particular unit or with a particular population.
- *Context*: In concert with the literature, the need exists for this project in a specific population and setting. This need can be reasonably described.
- *Possible methods*: Quality-improvement models/strategies and protocol implementation and evaluation approaches will be typical. You can gain experience with quality-improvement-type projects, change projects, or case study approaches.
- *Further reading*: Review books and resources on quality improvement, case study, and change theory.
- *Examples*: These projects might include implementing and testing an established protocol for pain management with patients with dementia. Or you might implement and test a communication protocol in a long-term care setting (see proposal abstract—Appendix H).

Why Evidence-Generating Approaches?

You have reviewed the evidence and found limited data on your problem or area of interest. For example, related to an increase in patient falls on the unit, you note that most protocols focus on internal patient factors relevant to falls rather than extrinsic room-safety issues. You believe that an observation survey or interview is needed to gain new evidence and help raise staff awareness about this issue. This might involve generating new-evidence resources. Nurses are often first to identify new challenges in patient care. Often this is where the need for further data originates. Projects will be identified as questions are asked to gain subject perceptions of a problem, knowledge about a problem, or perceived behaviors. Data-collection methods, including observation and document review, can also provide new data to help understand a problem. Box 10.3 summarizes this approach.

> **BOX 10.3**
>
> **Quick Outline: Proposing an Evidence-Generating Project**
>
> - *Current evidence*: If you find limited research literature specific to your topic and ask questions such as: Is my topic or problem area one that is new or unique in a selected area? Is this an area that has little evidence available to better understand or guide work with the problem? Is there more need for evidence in the practice world?
> - *Context*: In concert with the literature, the need exists for this project in a specific population and setting. This need can be reasonably described.
> - *Possible methods*: Strategies to gain basic knowledge/information on a topic from a selected population are diverse. Often you will consider basic descriptive study methods for this project. Sometimes the project may be framed as part of a quality-improvement project. For collecting evidence on a given problem, you might use tools such as needs surveys, environmental scans, guided discussion groups, observation tools, or simple interviews or surveys.
> - *Further readings*: Readings from quality-improvement and research texts specific to basic descriptive projects are useful.
> - *Examples*: If you find nursing assistants in long-term care are frustrated and uncomfortable with palliative care, you might seek evidence to better understand the problem. You might have a guided discussion or collect surveys as to their challenges and strategies in providing end-of-life palliative care. Or, if you are interested in rural health clinics, your approach might include surveying rural nurses about their strategies for managing a rural health population (see proposal abstract—Appendix F).

• • •

ADDITIONAL APPROACHES TO GUIDE THE EVIDENCE-BASED PROJECT

You have reviewed the literature and considered the quality of evidence available for your project. You have just reviewed three common approaches to clinical projects and are determining what might be most useful to you. Selecting from other common scholarly approaches may also be beneficial. These approaches, sometimes considered big-picture frameworks, can guide your proposal and be integrated along with the evidence-based approaches. It is interesting to note that often there is an overlap in methods used within each of these approaches. Framework examples include quality-improvement and change models, needs assessments, surveys, and other approaches.

Quality-Improvement and Change Models

As discussed in Chapter 4, quality improvement involves addressing a pressing clinical issue in terms of solving a problem or improving care. Improvement projects are planned to help promote safe clinical care delivery, interpersonal care aspects, and life quality. Typically, the scope is narrow, and the context is a specified unit or setting. Quality-improvement projects make a case for project need. The project integrates appropriate use of literature/best evidence with real-world practice, that is, articulation of how chart (electronic record review) data from your practice setting match an ideal evidence-based clinical pathway. It can help with articulation of problems leading to less-than-quality care or excess resource use. For example, in a large primary care setting with numerous doctors seeing one another's patients, the problem of consistency in treating patients with the new diagnosis of chronic lung disease could be mapped out using this process.

In another example, you notice the aging of your patient population and the increasing incidence of dementia. Staff seem to lack awareness of how best to communicate with these patients. One strategy will be to assess/confirm this need for staff improvement, identify and implement an evidence-based communication protocol, and evaluate the impact. Population and system issues can be addressed with these quality-improvement-type approaches.

Change projects typically use a traditional change model to guide the project. As part of a plan for a new evidence-based protocol on infection control, a model would guide one in naming the change plan, determining phases for implementation, considering potential barriers as well as facilitators, and determining how to evaluate outcomes. Goals are to minimize the barriers and focus on the facilitators. You will consider these potential challenges and strategies as part of your proposal. Involving staff in this process is a typical consideration in change models. This approach could build on the noted quality model, with additional focus on staff involvement.

Evaluation is also a component of these models. Naming the outcomes to be evaluated (i.e., pain-management improvements) and how these will be measured are key. Additional chapters in this text, including Chapters 8 and 12, further address tools that can be used in evaluation. Evaluation projects include generating evaluation questions, determining standards for effectiveness, designing evaluation tools, designating participants, collecting data, analyzing, and reporting (Fink, 2014).

Needs Assessments, Descriptive Surveys, and Interviews

As noted, diverse project approaches can relate to quality improvement and/or generate further evidence about a topic. Selected approaches that may be used to help frame a project or generate new information include needs assessments and descriptive surveys/interviews. Although an overview of these approaches is provided, once project decisions are made, further related references will be needed in guiding the project development.

Needs Assessments

Needs assessments, as introduced in Chapter 4, help provide the context for a project and are key project components. These can be very extensive, detailed projects in themselves, or practical assessments made primarily with available data, to show need for quality improvement. Needs assessments provide the opportunity to gain new data to help clarify a problem or help generate evidence about gaps in practices that currently exist. These are often the first step in a larger project, such as a new program in a community or hospital. Sometimes a systems model helps frame a needs assessment, that is, asking questions to determine structures and processes that currently exist and then considering how the new proposed program could build on or add to this. For example, a clinical problem in a long-term care setting might include older adult resident challenges, such as not eating well in a group dining setting. A further developed needs assessment gained from either formal or informal interviews and observations with staff and residents could help document the problem in greater detail. Paired with a review of the literature, a needs assessment helps to understand the who, what, and when of a problem. The literature provides the broad picture and the needs assessment helps focus the problem to a local context.

Questions to address in a needs assessment:

- Who/what are the people, the places, and process factors important in your future project?
- How have key needs of this entity been determined?
- How does the proposed project fit with the organization or community's goals?

Descriptive Surveys or Interviews and Related Approaches

These projects can help document participants' knowledge, behaviors, perceptions, or satisfaction specific to designated topics. An example would be surveying staff on knowledge about emerging research or soliciting their concerns about implementing/changing to a new staffing system. Designing small clinical projects that generate evidence can then provide the basis for learning about an issue and can be an important step in further developing larger projects.

Other Approaches

Case Studies

Case studies are another way to frame quality-improvement or evaluative clinical projects in one setting. A case study involves one specific unit, or perhaps one unique patient. In some situations multiple case studies are completed and compared. Case studies can be used to illustrate a problem; consider an approach for solving the problem; or address the need for different clinical approaches, theory applications, or further research. Learning about one family member's perceptions of long years of caregiving for a patient with late-stage Alzheimer's disease is one example of this approach (W. Bonnel, 1996). These projects can suggest strategies for better understanding care needs and generating potential strategies for further testing.

● ● ●

PROJECT MAPPING: THE BIG PICTURE

Back to the Project Triangle

Although proposal components are addressed in separate chapters of this book, there is an interplay among them; components are interrelated, and all are needed for completeness and wholeness of the project. This chapter lays out a sampling of approaches/methods to help organize the project plan. Part of this process is clearly aligning the project purpose with the proposed outcomes and methods as depicted in the project triangle.

A broad map saves one from problems down the road if links are made in the project triangle early on. Reviewing the project triangle along with literature and theory can help you identify where attention is needed on the project. Project questions to begin proposal deliberations have been noted earlier in this chapter and serve here as a reminder in project mapping: What is the available evidence on your topic? What is the product/process that you will package?

What broad approaches may be most helpful in gaining a better understanding and direction or guidance for your project? Further examples follow.

For example, as an advanced practice nurse (APN) in your hospital's occupational health department, you identify many staff who have problems with excess weight (and you are concerned with how this leads to further health problems and safety issues as well as providing poor role models for patients).

The need has been identified. This is a time for questions:

- Is there an evidence-based protocol available to implement (for helping staff)?
- If not, is there reasonable evidence in the literature that could be synthesized into a protocol?
- Is further evidence needed that could be gained from surveys or interviews with staff?
- What is the best direction for a project proposal?

The same approach could be used if, as an APN, you have identified a need for further resources to offer caregivers of patients with dementia.

- Is there an evidence-based protocol available to implement to help caregivers?
- If not, is there reasonable evidence in the literature that could be synthesized into a protocol?
- Is further evidence needed that could be gained from surveys or interviews with caregivers?
- What is the best direction for a project proposal?

As you begin to map your proposal plan further, early questions for each of the aforementioned examples will include:

- What theories or models have relevance to the situation you are trying to improve? Perhaps the health belief model or the health promotion model in the first case? A relevant theory on caregiving for the second?
- Will the ideas you are generating lead to a project with important implications or have potential for practice, education, and research?

As your project plans mature, further questions you will ask include: Is the project feasible? Is it effective and efficient in terms of cost and staff time? Is it acceptable to persons involved such as patients, staff, and providers?

Fundamental to all is that these questions keep the three points of the project triangle (purpose, methods, outcomes) aligned.

* * *

FURTHER CONSIDERATIONS FOR THE PROJECT-PROPOSAL MAP

Adding Further Details

Initially a work in progress, the project map helps fill in the details. It helps answer important project questions such as who, what, when, and where? Now that you have narrowed your problem, placed it in the context of the literature, and considered sample strategies to frame your clinical project, you are ready to brainstorm your more detailed project plan. As you reviewed this chapter, what approaches described could be effective and efficient in addressing your specified problem? What are the broad strategies you might use to map approaches to the problem/topic?

Continue detailing your proposed project plan with additional questions. This work in progress moves forward to a detailed plan and serves as a communication tool with colleagues/mentors and later guides in writing the proposal. As you move to the next decisions with your proposal, sample issues will include the following.

If you go with an evidence implementation/evaluation or evidence-generating-type project:

- Who will be the subjects (or the sample from your population)?
- What will be the setting?
- What specific outcomes are being sought?
- What are best methods for collecting data to evaluate?
- What will be an appropriate protocol or guidelines for the project?

If you go with an evidence synthesizing plus project, you are reviewing articles to summarize the best evidence on a topic.

- Although articles are not exactly subjects, you will talk about the numbers and type of articles, and how they were gathered.
- Sample questions to consider would be: What criteria will you use for article selection? What types of articles are acceptable? What review criteria will be used?
- What will be your methods for completing the search?
- What is your plan for the "plus" component? An evidence checklist? An evidence protocol for further testing?

Is Your Project Feasible?

The feasibility of your project will further determine your proposal methods. *Feasibility* refers to the project being practical or doable. Create a feasibility checklist for completing the project. Some of the following items can help make a case for feasibility and may also belong in your proposal appendix.

- Detailed work plan and timelines
- Summary of any needed resources and how they will be obtained
- Summary of needed competencies for completing the project and how they are attained
- Access to people, facilities, and situations, including any needed permissions
- Procedure approvals from human subjects committees/institutional review boards (Krathwohl & Smith, 2005)

● ● ●

TOOLS TO HELP: FURTHER MAPPING AND OUTLINING

Further mapping involves making the points of the project triangle all mesh/intertwine. Sample tools for brainstorming include visual tools and problem-solving approaches, templates, and writing tools. Decision trails are discussed as an important tool for documenting your project-proposal choices.

Visual Maps and Problem-Solving Models

For those who benefit from a visual perspective, create a visual diagram for what you want to happen. Concept maps are common approaches used for this. For those who think in a more linear fashion, additional approaches to help do this include flow diagrams and linear models.

Use of a problem-solving model, such as the basic nursing process, can help map plans as well. Questions to consider when mapping:

- Assess: Have you assessed the need for the project?
- Plan: Have you planned tentative methods?
- Implement: Have you considered potential challenges with implementation?
- Evaluation: Have you addressed a project evaluation plan?

Reflection, Writing, and Documenting

Reflective Writing

Continuation of your reflective writing allows you to self-assess and address your concerns or satisfaction with the project's progress (i.e., noting what still needs to be accomplished as well as highlighting the major accomplishments). Guided reflection can enhance self-evaluation of plans. It can lead to further questions and thoughts for the proposal.

Templates, Filling in the Spaces

Templates provide a type of framework with reminders for each project component. The visual cues help get all pieces and reminders needed to flow together. Consider using a one-page table and filling in the pieces there. A project template is provided in Appendix 10.1 using the Room Safety Scan Project (M. Bonnel, 2012) as a simple example.

Decision Trail

A decision trail provides a summary of important activities that have been completed in the process of developing the project (think of this as almost a type of recipe that allows others to see the process/activities you have used in developing your clinical project). This should be specific so that if others choose, they could replicate your procedures in another setting. Another way to think about the decision trail is as a listing by dates of specific activities you have completed for the project. This is sometimes referred to as an *audit trail*.

Project Mapping: Common Challenges to Avoid

Project mapping and troubleshooting include addressing common practical concerns during the planning phase. Use the following to help think about potential issues with your project during project planning.

- Is it the right-sized project—not too large or small?
- Is this the right time and place to address this issue? Are you or your team adequately prepared to take on the project?
- Are there any political issues or legal considerations in the proposed project setting that might impact project implementation?
- Do the points of the project triangle mesh? For example, matching methods, such as data to be collected, with the project purpose and planned outcomes.
- Are plans too broad or not adequately detailed for others to follow or replicate?

- Will the setting be challenging to access?
- Do you (the project director) have adequate background to carry out the project activities?
- Are plans to use selected equipment or resources realistic (Leedy & Omrod, 2013)?

Also learn from the experience of doctor of nursing practice (DNP) students who have preceded you in writing project proposals. Their advice is presented in the following box.

● ● ●

ADVICE FROM DNP STUDENTS

Project Mapping
Think about the big picture
- The proposal is like a huge jigsaw puzzle. Everything has to fit perfectly together or it does not work. Changing even a small study component can result in a totally different focus for a project.

Diagram, in the most basic and simple format, what needs to happen
- I am learning how to take a project idea and attempt to distill it down to the most basic elements for the project.

Use initial work to generate more questions
- The more I read, the more questions I have.

Discuss with others
- Interaction with others is helpful in that it highlights aspects of the project that you might not have thought about.
- Learning from my colleagues as they developed their project ideas was captivating.

Use your decision trail
- My decision trail, or paper trail, has been more than beneficial. It helps to identify where I have been and my trajectory along the path toward my accomplishments. It has prevented me from redoing a task or revisiting a problem.

SUMMARY

We have all had experience with maps. In the clinical project, the purpose statement is the project's clear destination. Now the intent is to find the best way (among multiple routes) to reach that destination. Mapping out the big picture of your project helps maintain the desired direction. You have identified your problem and the literature surrounding this problem. You have started to address the context or setting and population issues. Considering the project triangle, what approach seems the best match? As your project ideas come together, use techniques from this chapter to map out plans that can guide your project.

WEBSITES FOR FURTHER REVIEW

More ideas for mapping can be gained by reviewing resources at select websites such as national reports from the Academy of Sciences and the Agency for Healthcare Research and Quality (AHRQ). Ideas for small-scale projects might be gained from the following as well as similar national reports.

- *Improving Diagnosis in Healthcare* (2015): This report on preventing diagnostic errors includes toolkits such as best practices for improving communication:
  nationalacademies.org/hmd/~/media/Files/Report%20Files/
  2015/Improving-Diagnosis/DiagnosticError_Toolkit.pdf
- *Making Eye Health a Population Health Imperative: Vision for Tomorrow:*
  www.nap.edu/catalog/23471/making-eye-health-a-population-health
  -imperative-vision-for-tomorrow
- *AHRQ Fall Prevention Toolkit* (2013):
  www.ahrq.gov/sites/default/files/publications/files/fallpxtoolkit.pdf

NEXT CHAPTER UP

As discussed in this chapter, you are working on a big picture or map of your project proposal. The next chapter helps add the additional detail of more specific methods to use. In general, this includes data-collection tools (often from research or quality-improvement methods) and strategies that assist in implementing and evaluating your project. Remember that although components of each of the proposal chapters are addressed separately, there is an interplay among all components; each piece is needed to create a complete, cohesive project.

LEARNING ACTIVITIES

To-Do List

1. Finalize the literature review for best evidence on my topic of interest.
2. Determine the type and quality of literature that exists for my problem of interest.
3. Create a possibilities reflection (see the following learning activity).
4. Begin mapping my plan through a project template.

Possibilities Reflection

Reflective writing can often help better determine a map of possibilities for detailing a project about a specific problem/topic. Reflecting on possibilities might include the following:

- To learn more about my problem/topic, I might observe the following activities/situations: _____.
- I might talk to the following people: _____.
- I might review the following documents/resources: _____.
- Various ways to address this problem/topic from a project-methods perspective would include: _____.
- The most reasonable way to address this problem/topic from a project-methods perspective would be: _____.

_____

_____

_____

_____

_____

_____

REFERENCES

Academic Center for Evidence-Based Practice. (2013). ACE Star Model of knowledge transformation. Retrieved from http://www.acestar.uthscsa.edu/acestar -model.asp

Bonnel, M. (2012). *The room safety scan project.* Unpublished manuscript, Department of Nursing, Fort Hays State University, Hays, KS.

Bonnel, W. (1996). Not gone and not forgotten, a spouse's experience of late stage Alzheimer's disease caregiving. *Journal of Psychosocial Nursing, 34*(8), 23–27.

Fink, A. (2014). *Evaluation fundamentals: Insights into the outcomes, effectiveness, and quality of health programs* (3rd ed.). New York, NY: Sage.

Krathwohl, D., & Smith, N. (2005). *How to prepare a dissertation proposal: Suggestions for students in education and the social and behavioral sciences.* Syracuse, NY: Syracuse University Press.

Leedy, P., & Omrod, J. (2013). *Practical research: Planning and design* (10th ed.). Boston, MA: Pearson.

Melnyk, B. M., & Fineout-Overholt, E. (2014). *Evidence-based practice in nursing & healthcare: A guide to best practice* (3rd ed.). Philadelphia, PA: Wolters Kluwer/ Lippincott Williams & Wilkins.

10.1

EVIDENCE-BASED-PROJECT TEMPLATE

The following provides a template to begin mapping your project ideas; a completed template example of an evidence-based project (EBP) follows.

Title of EBP Project				
Problem Summary		Current Best Evidence		
Purpose Statement		Proposed Project Design What Theory Will Guide the Project?		
What data will be collected?	What tools will be used to collect this data?	What is the quality of the measure?	Who will collect the data? How will the data-collection methods be systematic and rigorous?	How will the data be analyzed?

EXAMPLE: EVIDENCE GENERATING

Title of EBP Project: Room Safety Scan	
Problem Summary *Patient falls in clinical setting are a major problem. Literature review suggests intrinsic patient factors are better understood than extrinsic factors.*	Current Best Evidence *Although literature summarizing intrinsic patient factors leading to falls is evident, limited data are found about the extent of environmental issues leading to falls.*
Purpose Statement *Purpose: To raise awareness of fall-safety issues by systematically observing patient rooms for the presence of environmental safety issues.*	Proposed Paper/Project Design *Descriptive observational project to promote improved quality care.*
	What Theory Will Guide the Project? *Broad systems theory guides attention to structure and process of care to prevent fall outcomes.*

(continued)

What data will be collected? *Safety factors in 30 occupied patient rooms.*	What tools will be used to collect this data? *Room safety observation checklist.*	What is the quality of the measure? *New tool developed from the literature. Peer review to be completed.*	Who will collect the data? How will the data-collection methods be systematic and rigorous? *Project director will collect data over three weekends.*	How will the data be analyzed? *Descriptive statistics for each safety item and scores as a whole will be reported.*

Source: Bonnel (2012).

11

Writing the Methods Section: Organizing the Advanced Clinical Project Proposal

Reflective Questions

In Chapter 10, you considered the importance of mapping out broad plans for your proposal. The following reflective questions help you consider further development of your methods section and organize learning for this chapter. With which of the following are you most comfortable?

- What makes detailing proposal methods important?
- What specific methods are addressed in the proposal?
- What specific approaches could work for your project?

• • •

THE IMPORTANCE OF THE METHODS SECTION

This chapter helps identify the big picture regarding research and/or quality-improvement methods for your project. A function of the methods section is to address what you plan to do and why you plan to do that. The methods section describes the process that will be used to gain the project product or outcomes. Once you move beyond synthesizing the evidence, if you are proposing an evidence-generating or evidence-testing approach for your project, the following elements need to be described:

- *Setting*: Specify elements of the specific setting in your project.
- *Population*: Specify the population you will study, giving at least a broad description of participants.
- *If intervention is to be used*: Describe the intervention and its component parts in sufficient detail that others could reproduce it; outline initial plans for how the intervention is to be implemented.
- *Data collection*: Describe the specific data-collection plan.

While the previous discussion addressed evidence-testing and evidence-generating approaches, the "evidence synthesis plus" is a bit different. Since the initial focus in the evidence synthesis plus project is the literature review, further planning points will depend on your "plus." As indicated, this may relate to using the evidence synthesis to develop checklists to be used for chart review, specific protocol development from the evidence, or other quality improvement approaches.

Writing a project proposal incorporates many components. Key in aligning these components is the project triangle. This chapter focuses on the methods point of the triangle and helps address "how do I do the methods?"

* * *

FOCUSING THE PROJECT METHODS

Project methods will vary depending on the project approach you choose. Let's say you are working with patients with Parkinson's disease (PD) and want to develop a project related to support groups for those patients. In this example, the assessment of your population, potential settings, and the literature suggest the benefit of a descriptive or evidence-generating project.

If you had a strong evidence base or protocol for a needed topic in your clinical setting, perhaps swallowing problems in patients with late-stage PD, you might decide to implement and evaluate a new protocol, a type of intervention, with your staff. When intervention is to be used in your project, you will outline initial plans for how the intervention is to be implemented. Describe the intervention and its component parts in sufficient detail so that others could reproduce it. For example, Standards for Quality Improvement Reporting Excellence (SQUIRE; 2015) quality-improvement project guidelines address components to include in your planning such as who will implement the intervention (individual or multiple), and what are their qualifications (or the methods needed to train them)? Any issues concerning internal validity of the project intervention and plans for monitoring the fidelity of the intervention should be described as thoroughly as possible. In addition to thoroughly describing the intervention plan, address the context as much as possible. This includes place factors (the health care/practice context) and people factors (patient-specific variables and staff type/amount of staffing) that are the background for the intervention protocol. Implementing and evaluating the protocol will also include monitoring data-collection plans, as described in the following.

As you read through this chapter, continue to refer to Box 11.1 and think about the initial challenges presented in project planning. Note similarities and differences between this project and the one you are working on.

BOX 11.1

Methods Questions: Parkinson's Disease (PD) Online Support Group Example

If you were working with patients with PD and were concerned about their emotional-support issues, what are some of the problems/issues that come to mind? What are some potential responses by health care providers? What might lead to a project to help address identified need? Your response, of course, is to head to the literature to gain answers. You will have to first review the literature to determine best evidence for support groups as a resource. That will include a review of evidence specifically for patients with PD. What questions might come to mind?

- Based on the evidence available, should you recommend support groups or are further questions raised? What do you still need to know?
- Does your evidence address the changing needs of patients who are progressing through the disease? Does the literature cover all disease stages, or are there special needs for patients with later stages of the disease or at early stages of the disease?
- Does your literature address the setting/access/context for support groups? Does the literature address advancing PD and online versus face-to-face group strategies/challenges?
- If you find there is little evidence in the literature on PD patients and support-group issues, what are your options for framing a project? Would you be more likely to work with early-stage or later stage patients? Would you be more likely to consider a descriptive project, gaining patient perspectives, or a protocol evaluating a specific type of support group?

• • •

PLANS FOR GAINING EVALUATION DATA

Plans for gaining data provide one of the most interesting parts of the project proposal. It is here that you devise plans to organize information/evidence in new ways to learn new things about a topic. This is central to clinical scholarship. To make sure you have good data to share, you need good methods for data collection. Approaches to be considered in this chapter include (a) interview/survey, (b) observations, and (c) document or electronic record reviews. A reminder of these approaches, from your previous coursework, is provided in quick summary format in Table 11.1.

Another way to think about this, is that as you generate the methods section of your proposal, you will have to describe tools that help you gain data/evidence to best solve your problem. For example, nursing process is a problem-solving model that reminds one to assess for need, name the problem, plan the project response, implement, and then evaluate. Consider what approaches to data collection (interview, observation, and record review) can best help gain data to address your project purpose and proposed outcomes. Both qualitative and quantitative approaches to using these tools are also considered.

Methods for Gaining Data: The Project Triangle

Making the methods choices fit with the project purpose and desired project outcomes is the goal. Recall the project triangle (see Appendix A), in which the purpose, methods, and outcomes represent the three points. Any inconsistency among the three will make the triangle fall apart, as the three lines won't match up into the shape of a triangle. Therefore, a key aspect is keeping those three components—purpose, methods, and outcomes—in alignment with one another.

The purpose statement will be based on the problem and current evidence found in the literature, and provides the basis for an evidence-generating, synthesizing, or implementing/testing-type project. Again, there needs to be consistency among the purpose, methods, and outcomes you choose for your project.

In going back to the project triangle, your project purpose also dictates the types of methods needed for a complete/quality project. Ask: What has the purpose statement promised? What are the intended outcomes? This guides choices for data collection and sampling. For example, when you plan to collect project data, you will be making choices about interviews, surveys, observations, document reviews, or some combination thereof.

Gaining Project Data Through Selected Tools

How can that data best be gained? Consider broad choices and then further detail can be added later. Common tools for gaining project data are described, including interview, survey, observation, and/or document-review opportunities (as well as determining the best qualitative or quantitative approaches to use). Once broad choices are made, prepare a more detailed plan (negotiating the best tools/approaches) while keeping in mind the practical resources available are all considerations in planning your methods. You want to use the best methods possible to get the best results because even one weak piece can lead to a weak project.

● ● ●

WHICH METHODS FOR DATA COLLECTION WOULD WORK BEST?

The project purpose you choose influences the methods you use. For example, if your purpose is to generate evidence on a new clinical challenge, then you might choose either a qualitative or quantitative survey approach to gain data about that challenge. As you recall, within the qualitative or quantitative paradigms, various common data-collection methods include interviews, surveys, observation, or document reviews. The paradigm you chose should guide the more specific methods chosen. For example, if the qualitative approach is chosen, then the qualitative theme guides throughout. In other words, written surveys or interview prompts are primarily open ended or use a basic descriptive format. Quantitative approaches would use a more structured survey or interview approach with numeric responses/rating scales.

The following paragraphs first consider qualitative versus quantitative approaches to methods. Then common tools used within both qualitative and quantitative paradigms (interviews, surveys, observations, and document reviews) are discussed.

Qualitative Context: Issues to Consider

The qualitative paradigm considers the world through a lens of openness and complexity. The value of broad open-ended questions directed by qualitative paradigms includes gaining perspectives from the subject about his or her perceived knowledge, attitudes, and behaviors. Qualitative methods typically include gaining some type of word data, as opposed to numeric data. Content analysis for common themes is typically used with themes summarizing the data reported.

Qualitative methods provide a beginning toolkit for gaining data that can be authentic and meaningful. Well-known qualitative tools, such as interview and observation, bring real-world experiences to life through the written word and provide descriptive richness for data sharing. Qualitative data can help describe and make a compelling case for work in early descriptive stages. It can serve as the basic descriptive data for sharing and developing future projects. Qualitative methods capture word themes that convey experiences in a richer texture than quantitative numbers alone.

Benefits of qualitative methods include gaining subjects' true understandings from their perspectives. A depth of understanding missing from numerical summaries can be gained. Typically, a small sample size will be beneficial in learning about others' experiences, for example, interviews of those new to a role like geriatric nurse practitioner (Bonnel, Belt, Hill, Wiggins, & Ohm, 2000). Sample approaches include broad open-ended interviews either with individuals or with groups. Qualitative projects can also include surveys with broad open-ended questions or use broad observation guides for a specific setting or population. Qualitative approaches also provide opportunities to make broad observations such as windshield surveys or "walk-throughs" of new or unique settings. Theory or models from community or public health or organizational leadership coursework can provide examples for strategies to organize these initial observations.

Challenges to qualitative approaches include the small sample sizes used, which often limit the ability to generalize the findings. These are typically descriptive projects that do not focus on testing hypotheses. Often, approaches are used to study new topics or areas with limited research. They are often used for projects that are evidence generating. They are also used to gain qualitative perspectives in evaluative projects.

Quantitative Context: Issues to Consider

The quantitative paradigm is considered to be focused and deterministic; often this approach is compared to a closed system. Quantitative approaches are used to capture and summarize knowledge, attitudes, or behaviors. This involves using tools to gain numerical data representing these qualities, as opposed to word data. These tools provide an opportunity to gain data that can help one understand the numerical qualities of an attribute. Surveys and other tools for observation and document review help specify through numbers what is going on or enable the researcher to make comparisons.

A challenge to this method is finding measures or survey instruments that truly capture the concepts being studied. Quantitative approaches lose the richness of descriptive themes gained with qualitative methods but have the benefit of more easily conveying or comparing numerical data about diverse groups.

Quantitative approaches can also help describe and make a compelling case for work in early descriptive stages. Quantitative methods capture numeric summaries that promote ease of comparison. Quantitative approaches help summarize large groups of responses more easily than qualitative themes. A quantitative approach is often useful in data collection for projects that involve implementing and evaluating a new protocol.

* * *

STRATEGIES FOR COLLECTING/GAINING DATA

Qualitative and quantitative paradigms provide the broad context or background assumptions for the choices you make in gaining data. These paradigms set the stage for the more detailed data-collection plan (to learn about the problem or topic of interest). How many ways are there to collect data? To keep things simple, broad approaches of interview/survey, observation, and record review (i.e., charts or electronic health records [EHRs]) are discussed. Further choices and detail then need to be added to each. Information about these common tools for gaining project data follows.

Interviews and Surveys

Interviews and surveys provide an opportunity to gain information about peoples' knowledge, attitudes, or perceived behaviors. Interview guides and surveys can be developed from either qualitative or quantitative perspectives. Qualitative methods more typically use open-ended questions with verbal responses. Quantitative approaches are more typically closed-ended questions seeking some type of response with numerical coding potential.

- *Face-to-face, individual interviews*: These provide an opportunity to converse with an individual about a specific topic, typically to gain others' perceptions. They include the value of engaging in nonverbal communication about the topic/questions. Opportunities to extend questions and generate follow-up responses to questions that emerge can be valuable.

- *Face-to-face, group interviews*: These provide the benefit of gaining individuals' thoughts on a topic. They also provide further opportunity to stimulate ideas from others with brainstorming-type approaches to gain ideas/topics individuals may not have thought to share. Challenges may be to make sure the investigator receives a true opinion versus "group think."

Written Surveys

Written surveys provide the opportunity to learn from others' knowledge or experience related to a topic. They can be easy to administer, but a disadvantage they share is they offer no opportunity to follow up or clarify why the individual responded as he or she did. Also, much piloting work is required to make sure participants interpret and respond as the investigator intends.

Planning for Interviews or Surveys

When considering interviews or surveys, basic decisions include: Are well-developed tools available? Are these appropriate qualitative or quantitative approaches? Do they define the concepts of interest in the same way as your project does? Tool descriptions are further addressed in Chapters 12 and 13.

You also need to plan and be very specific in your proposal regarding the actual strategies you will use in completing the interviews or surveys. For example, what will be the context or setting for the written, or face to face, data collection? Where will this happen? Will there be privacy if this is a sensitive subject? Will there be an opportunity to collect data during a scheduled clinic waiting time or before a class? How will participants return these forms to you? Online surveys are another consideration. They add to the speed of data collection as long as participants can easily access and have motivation to complete the survey.

Observations

Observation allows opportunity to view activities in natural settings (Warren & Karner, 2005). Observation provides an opportunity to learn new information or confirm concepts and processes. Observations have value in learning about situations, competencies, and behaviors. Observing classrooms or clinical agencies, the investigator learns about roles, practices, and strategies of people they observe and also gain information about the setting's structure and processes. Observations may be used less frequently than surveys and interviews, but they are valuable in learning about real-life behaviors.

Specifying or mapping out and documenting a plan that includes time or event factors to observe allows better opportunity to capture what is intended. For example, in an early project, Bonnel (1993), using a qualitative format, completed an observation of a group dining experience for long-term-care residents; a very detailed plan for observations included length of time, the observer's role, and specific schedule of observations. Observation data can also be collected in more structured settings like skills labs. Hober (2012), for example, observed students' experiences in a simulation lab to seek concepts of clinical judgment as part of the simulation. Clinical lab observations also provide opportunities related to staff development and competency assessment.

Record or Document Reviews

A common data-collection strategy, especially in quality improvement, has always been chart reviews. This is a nonintrusive strategy for collecting data. Although typically this was done on hard copies of charts, EHRs have now emerged.

EHRs have changed the way chart reviews are done and provide many advantages. Speed of review is one. Fairly rapidly, these tools provide collections of data that would have taken hours to access and review in the past. It is important to remember that just as chart-review projects included a data-collection sheet, the electronic equivalent of this sheet is still required. Random questions of the data will not meet the project needs. You will need to give thought to how you structure your electronic "data-collection" guide.

Chart reviews can also provide challenges to data collection. Challenges or disadvantages to EHRs, and other forms of written record review, include that the clinician/researcher has no control over the data that were collected. For example, if you are reviewing care processes, there may be inaccuracies in the recording; that is, something might have actually been done but not charted. Or, if physiologic measures such as blood pressures are gained (usually fairly strong credible measures), there is no control over the protocol used in gaining these measures. Also, there is no ability to ask further questions about missing data.

Advantages or benefits of electronic records data include reasonable access to clinical data that can help answer, in particular, quality-improvement questions. Large electronic databases, such as the National Database of Nursing Quality Indicators, also exist, and may be valuable in collecting meaningful data for specified project purposes.

● ● ●

ADDITIONAL COMMENTS ON DATA COLLECTION

Again, for each data-collection method (interview, survey, observation, and record review), there are many variations related to the structure of items. This includes, for example, highly structured questions through the quantitative paradigm as well as the open-ended structure of the qualitative paradigm. In some cases diverse methods can also be combined in useful/appropriate ways, providing a type of triangulation. A good research text can provide further detail to guide additional decisions. With all cases of collecting data, addressing appropriate human subjects and Health Insurance Portability and Accountability Act (HIPAA) guidelines are required as discussed in Chapter 14.

Table 11.1 provides sample approaches to these common data-collection tools. Each of these tools can be considered from both qualitative and quantitative perspectives. As you review, consider how many ways there are to use each

TABLE 11.1

DATA-COLLECTION TOOLS

Samples used in interviews, surveys, observations, and reviews include:

Tool	Sample Approaches	Your Examples?
Surveys	Face-to-face written survey Email or traditional mail Electronic survey	
Interviews	Personal face to face Group guided discussions	
Observation	Clinical labs Clinical setting Public settings	

of these; this is the fun part. Consider also how each might (or might not) be relevant to the project you are planning.

* * *

PROJECT TRIANGLE EXAMPLES

Remember that whatever method you chose must allow alignment of the points of the project triangle. Purpose, methods, and outcomes need to support each other. Project triangle examples, specific to evidence-generating and evidence-testing methods, follow.

Evidence Generating

- *Purpose*: To determine need for an onsite health clinic at a large assisted-living clinic
- *Methods*: Qualitative observations of setting (people and place factors); qualitative interviews with staff/residents about current processes and additional need
- *Seeking outcomes*: Needs assessment report that summarizes planning needs for an onsite clinic

Evidence Implementing and Testing

- *Purpose*: To determine success of a new evidence-based discharge protocol for patients with congestive heart failure (CHF)
- *Methods*: Qualitative/quantitative survey of patients and their family members on readiness for discharge; guided discussion with staff on challenges/strategies for using the protocol
- *Seeking outcomes*: Documentation of successful protocol or needed improvements

* * *

SAMPLE AND SETTING CONSIDERATIONS FOR YOUR PROPOSAL

Identifying clearly in your proposal the setting and the population your project will study are key to helping your reader gain context. Consider the following setting and population issues as you make these plans and write up these sections.

Clearly Describe the Setting

To describe the setting, you will specify elements of the specific setting in your project. For example, if you want to consider the benefits of "educational gaming" as a strategy for a clinical education-related problem in a large health care system, the education protocol could be placed in the context of all staff education, health-professions education, nursing-student education, or nursing-staff-development education. It could also be placed in the frame of one clinical unit, a large health care system, or systems across a state or the country. Clearly framing your setting (and sample) helps focus your project.

To describe this context or setting for your project, you might first create a big-picture description or "systems" perspective of the overall setting and then fill in the parts/details such as the relevant people factors, place factors, and process factors related to the issue or topic. For example, in a study of a particular long-term care unit, you might identify the types of rooms, the number of people in the setting, common unit activities, and other factors relevant to your project. You might address what makes this unit similar or different from others.

Clearly Describe Sampling Choices

As you address your project plans, determine whether there will be human subjects and who they will be. Address how any subjects will be selected to participate in your project. Making informed choices about potential subjects for data collection is an important proposal component. What populations or clinical entities will provide you the information you need? An entire population or selected subgroups? Once you have addressed these points, you will provide at least a broad description of the population of interest.

For example, related to the initial case interests with PD support groups for patients, varied considerations are needed to identify your population. Some of the descriptive components and questions related to the population of study should include:

- Who makes up the broad population of patients with PD in your region of interest?
- Who makes up the accessible population? Are there currently groups that involve patients in the beginning, middle, or late stages of the disease?
- Will these individuals be in groups that are online or face to face? Do the groups involve caregivers, families, or patients only (or a mix)? Are there other unique population factors that should be considered, for example, younger versus older patients?

Sampling Issues

Consider the different options in sampling choices and make the choices complementary to the methods chosen. For example, random sampling provides value in meeting assumptions for more sophisticated statistical procedures. In general, samples with larger numbers are more representative of the population of interest. Assumptions for quantitative statistics, for example, indicate at least an N of 30 to represent the population. Further discussions about quantitative statistics required for a project analysis are discussed in Chapter 12.

In qualitative projects, typically the convenience sample rules. In early descriptive stages of study, a small N is considered acceptable. Smaller numbers can still provide important descriptive information to help understand a topic or learn about populations' needs. For example, if you are asking rural nurses about challenges and approaches they use to best support patients in settings with scant resources, a sample size of 10 could provide good beginning descriptive data. A qualitative project can help describe and make a compelling initial case relevant to the problem.

How will your sampling choices relate to your projected outcomes and analysis? These choices play a major role in determining to whom the results of your project may be relevant. This applies, for example, if you want to make the case that your results have implications beyond your population sample and setting, in other words generalizing findings to another population or setting. In many clinical projects, you will describe as clearly as possible your methods and findings, but not have adequate control of variables to generalize these findings. If that is the case, your detailed project can still be useful to others who may wish to replicate your project and see whether similar outcomes are gained in their setting.

Making a good sampling choice will involve knowing your project plan, and the strengths/weaknesses of each approach. In addition, it is critical to consider whether the preferred approach is actually doable. Sometimes there are trade-offs between what is preferred and what is doable; you, as the project director, make the case for why you make the choices you make.

Quick Questions to Consider About Potential Sampling in Your Project

Ask yourself whether you have addressed each of the following:

- Is the population clearly defined?
- Is the population accessible?
- Are choices of convenience or random sampling justified?

- Are sampling procedures sufficiently detailed for replication?
- Are sampling choices appropriate to the purpose statement/project question?

• • •

SO, WHICH APPROACHES DO YOU USE FOR THE PROPOSAL?

This chapter talks broadly about methods. But which methods you choose will relate most closely to the type of clinical project design you focus on. As you consider your topic, think back to any similarities with the PD support group example. As described in Chapter 10, selected ways to use the best evidence for projects include:

Evidence-synthesis plus: Does literature/evidence exist about support groups that has not been synthesized for patients with PD? Would evidence lead to protocols for online groups or face-to-face groups? These could be possibilities.

Evidence testing: Does evidence exist in the form of a protocol for chronic care support groups that could be evaluated specifically for PD? Could the protocol be further validated as successful by participants or providers? These could be possibilities.

Evidence generating: Is more evidence needed related to specific concerns about groups for patients with PD? Could you ask clients in support groups their opinions? Could you ask clinical providers their opinions? Would possibilities exist for using interviews or surveys to gain further data? These could be possibilities.

Again, once the literature has been evaluated and a purpose statement determined, your project purpose will guide the methods you use. Within those larger paradigms of qualitative approaches and quantitative approaches, choices about surveys, interviews, observation, or document review will also be considered. Begin to map out the project triangle with appropriate methods to develop proposal plans. Guidance for the appropriate use of methods for the type of project you're conducting is developed with a mentor.

• • •

WRITING UP THE METHODS

Where and how does the methods section fit in the proposal? Scholarly proposals are typically arranged in sections that first include introductory materials, then the review of the literature, and third, the detailed methods section.

Within the methods section, the common scholarly "parts" noted in the following list can help organize your project methods. Describe specifically in your plan the following as part of your methods section:

- *Setting*: Specify elements of the specific setting in your project.
- *Population/Sampling*: How is the population defined (inclusion/exclusion criteria)?
- *Sampling*: Specify the population you will study giving at least a broad description.
- *Specific project implementation plans and evaluation methods*: Describe any intervention or procedure in fine detail. These strategies should be described in enough specific detail so that others could replicate the interventions or procedures you will use.

Creating a table of contents can serve as a helpful guide in organizing key components of the methods section. If you are in school as you complete your project, the school often has set guidelines for the specific headings to be completed for the proposal. If you are in a clinical agency with specific criteria to be addressed before submission to the Human Subjects Committee, that needs to be addressed as well. If yours is a clinical proposal to seek funding, funding agencies typically have outlined specified categories. Turning the guides into headings when possible helps the reader and typically improves the quality of the product. As previously noted, an abstract or two-page plan draft can keep the proposal tightly packaged for discussions and decision making by team members.

• • •
_____

PROJECT METHODS, QUICK QUESTIONS

If you are collecting data for your clinical project, does your proposal address each of the following?

- Does it have methods that fit the project purpose and proposed outcomes?
- Does it provide a description of the population and a strategy for sampling?
- Does it specify procedures for data collection?
- What is its timeline?
- Have you verified resource accessibility?
- Have you resolved any human subjects and institutional review board issues?

Also learn from the experience of doctor of nursing practice (DNP) students who have preceded you in developing project proposals. Their advice is presented in the following box.

• • •

ADVICE FROM DNP STUDENTS

Methods

Think about putting together the pieces of the proposal puzzle
- It is certainly like searching for detail after detail to fit each piece together.
- In retrospect, I should have spent more time looking for and reviewing similar projects to guide my thought process.

Go back to your textbooks
- Once you have a plan in mind, refocus on what your research text says about your particular plans (i.e., if you plan to use a descriptive survey, read more about that).

Focus on your specific methods
- Try to think methodically about each and every step for data collection.
- While reading, everything seems important to know, understand, and apply. Focus on the chapters or concepts that should get most of the attention.

Structure the methods
- Learn how to structure the methods section of a project proposal and the importance of being complete and thorough.

Be clear in your write-up of the methods section
- When writing a methods section, what seems clear the first several times you write out the details, probably isn't. Every time I came back to read my methods sections I realized it wasn't as clear as it seemed when I looked at it the time before. I was still tweaking the final product up until the moment I submitted the proposal. The devil is truly in the details.

SUMMARY

This chapter talks broadly about methods and choices for use in clinical project proposals. Qualitative and quantitative paradigms provide background for common data-collection choices of interviews, surveys, observations, and record reviews. The methods you choose will relate to the purpose and outcomes you plan to focus on. As noted, there are multiple approaches to these topics. Various choices keep clinical projects interesting and echo the importance of identifying early on exactly what you need and want to do.

WEBSITES FOR FURTHER REVIEW

When planning a methods section, keep returning to your project purpose. Examples of resources for gaining more ideas for methods sections can be gained by reviewing online examples and resources at select websites. See examples at the following websites.

- Qualitative resources—*Journal, The Qualitative Review*: nsuworks.nova.edu/tqr
- Quantitative evaluation sites—Informal Science/Evaluation www.informalscience.org/evaluation/evaluation-tools-instruments

Resources for gaining ideas for project protocols can also be gained by reviewing resources such as those provided by the Academy of Sciences. Ideas for small-scale projects might be gained from these and similar national reports.

- *Families Caring for an Aging America* (2016): This National Academy of Sciences report addresses family needs and challenges related to care-giving, as well as synthesizing successful interventions and outcomes: www.nationalacademies.org/hmd/Reports/2016/families-caring -for-an-aging-america.aspx

NEXT CHAPTER UP

As you consider approaches to data collection, you are also thinking ahead to how you will gain credible data. You will consider strategies for data collection that promote confidence in the tools chosen for your project and help to ensure that the resultant findings are reliable and valid.

LEARNING ACTIVITIES

Pulling Together Methods and Sampling, Case Example

Based on the readings, what strategies could you suggest to enhance sampling and project methods/approaches (dependable data, reasonable size project) for the following case?

In your hospital, you want to implement and evaluate an evidence-based strategy for communication tips to prevent agitated behaviors in residents with dementia. Which strategies are best to begin?

- A large hospital-wide program? Piloting/evaluating on one medical unit? Other choices?
- Who would you collect outcome data from? What type of data would you collect? What would be your methods for data collection?
- How could you set this plan up with the points of the project triangle (purpose, methods, and outcomes)?

Reflecting Further on Your Project Plans

- At this point, what seems to be reasonable and to work well for the plan you are considering?
- What other options might work as well?
- Address the pros and cons of each of your ideas. What will best meet your planned purpose? What will work best given your context and experience?

To-Do List

1. Complete further reading related to specific approaches you would like to use in your project. Look at examples of other projects that have been completed using similar methods.
2. Consider how you will best access the people or physical resources needed to complete your project.
3. Consider the "so what" or "why-this-is-important" factor related to your proposed plans.

REFERENCES

Bonnel, W. (1993). Managing the work of eating: The nursing home group dining experience. *Journal of Nutrition for the Elderly, 13*(1), 1–10.

Bonnel, W., Belt, J., Hill, D., Wiggins, S., & Ohm, R. (2000). Challenges and strategies for initiating a nursing facility practice. *Journal of the American Academy of Nurse Practitioners, 12*(9), 353–359.

Hober, C. (2012). *Student perceptions of the observer role play experiences in the implementation of a high fidelity patient simulation in bachelor's degree nursing programs* (Doctoral dissertation). Retrieved from http://kuscholarworks.ku.edu/dspace/bitstream/1808/9981/1/Hober_ku_0099D_11950_DATA_1.pdf

Standards for Quality Improvement Reporting Excellence. (2015). Revised standards for quality improvement reporting excellence, SQUIRE 2.0. Retrieved from http://www.squire-statement.org/index.cfm?fuseaction=Page.ViewPage&PageID=471

Warren, C., & Karner, T. (2005). *Discovering qualitative methods: Field research, interviews, and analysis.* Oxford, UK: Oxford University Press.

12

Gaining Credible Clinical
Project Data: Being
Systematic and Objective

Reflective Questions

Data collection is often a central component of clinical projects. In previous chapters, you considered the importance of developing broad data-collection plans for your project proposal. The following reflective questions help you consider further development of your methods section and organize learning for this chapter. As you make a plan for gaining the data, with which of the following are you most comfortable?

- Why is it important to address detailed plans for data collection?
- What procedures can help you make a plan that is systematic and objective?
- What strategies will you use to promote confidence in tools used and the resultant findings?

When writing a project proposal, addressing the quality of the data to be collected is central. This involves clearly describing the properties of the data-collection tools and identifying systematic, replicable protocols for data collection. Being systematic, objective, and using credible tools are key considerations. Also key is aligning these components in the project triangle. Building on the varied project plans previously described, this chapter focuses on further detailing the methods component of the project triangle. This builds on earlier discussions of qualitative and quantitative approaches to interviews, observations, and record reviews. Specific plans for collecting data in systematic, valid, and reliable ways are described in this chapter.

• • •

PROVIDING A DETAILED PLAN FOR DATA COLLECTION

It is helpful to first recall where the proposal-writing process has already taken you and the decisions made. This includes seeking data as part of the big picture of purpose, methods, and outcomes. With this information in mind, the big picture includes addressing the specific how, when, and what of data collection. The plan for collecting data should make clear statements about what data are to be collected and how that data will be collected. This chapter further addresses gaining data that are accurate, reliable, and meaningful as you move on to the specifics of data collection, addressing components that need to be addressed within your clinical project.

With Your Clinical Project in Mind

What qualitative or quantitative approaches or tools will you be using? How will you describe your tools and your protocols?

- For example, will you be using survey or interview questions that address factual knowledge, attitudes, and behaviors or questions that identify subjective states or perspectives?
- Or will you be using observations or document reviews to gain data about a specified concept/issue?

Once you decide how data will be collected in your project, you will be naming and clearly describing in your proposal both the tools to be used and the specific protocol or approaches to be followed that can support data accuracy and quality. The following paragraphs further detail how your proposal needs to describe the instruments for data collection and the protocol you will follow. The more complete and thorough the job you do now, in respect to proposed data-collection steps and anticipated problems, the easier the actual implementation of data collection will be later.

• • •

DESCRIBING CREDIBLE/TRUSTWORTHY TOOLS

For others to value your work, they need to understand how you have gained the data. You should describe the instruments used and the reliability and validity of these tools (Box 12.1). In describing the data-collection tools/instruments, at minimum it is necessary to:

- Share a thorough description of the tools
- Share any reliability and validity for the tools that have been reported in the literature

Share a Thorough Description

Name the tool you plan to use and describe briefly the historical development of the tool, including when and how it was developed. Describe examples of other projects that have used this tool. Include strengths and weaknesses of the tool. For example, if you are addressing "caring" approaches of critical care nurses, your survey could be a tool developed from Watson's work that addressed the 10 carative factors described in Watson's caring theory (Nelson & Watson, 2011). You would note that each of the 10 items has a 4-point range of 1 (low) to 4 (high). You would report this description and then provide examples of how other studies have used this tool. This would include further discussion of the tool's qualities, including reliability and validity. In addition, you would note this tool as consistent with the caring theory you chose to guide your study, including consistency with your project definitions of caring.

Share Reliability and Validity

Reliability and *validity* are common research terms. The approaches to reliability and validity vary, depending on the type of project to be done. The concept of reliability means methods are dependable or replicable, and the concept of validity means the methods are truthful representations of the data. In describing survey reliability, a common measure to note is internal consistency reliability, or Cronbach's alpha. This indicates how well or reliably the tool has "worked" in previous studies. Any concepts of validity described in the literature are also noted (such as construct- or criterion-related validity from previous work on the tool).

Sometimes when projects use qualitative tools, concepts of reliability and validity are described using alternate terms. For example, the term trustworthiness considers the concepts of credibility, dependability, and confirmability of qualitative data. Also, potential for transferablity of the project findings is considered (Polit & Beck, 2012).

BOX 12.1

DESCRIBING THE INSTRUMENTS

Example 1: Electronic Health Record Survey

For a simple survey, description might begin as follows: This project will use a survey consisting of both closed-ended responses and broad open-ended questions that were developed from items identified in the review of the literature. The questions for this descriptive survey included 12 questions. First, background questions about students' opinions are asked and then open-ended questions seeking further clarification of students' ideas are posed. This includes 10 structured-response questions (4-point rating) about electronic health records (EHRs) and two open-ended questions. Potential total scores for the 10 structured items range from 10 to 40 (high rating). The full questionnaire is provided in Appendix 12.1.

Example 2: Health Behaviors Survey

For a more developed survey, description might begin as follows: A tool developed by Walker, Sechrist, and Pender (1987), the Health Promoting Lifestyle Profile II, will be used to measure health behaviors. This is a 52-item scale that addresses five subscales of health, including physical activity, nutrition, health responsibility, stress management, and interpersonal relationships. The 52 items are answered with a 4-point response to indicate subjects' personal habits (never, sometimes, often, and routinely). The authors reported high internal consistency reliability, and construct validity was confirmed by factor analysis. Further studies have used this tool and also reported greater than .90 reliability.

Describe Related Credibility Issues

Further methods of assessing confirmability include the decision trail that you have already started to track your project decisions. As you recall, decision trails are objective progress records that document processes and decisions from project beginning to end. This is sometimes called an *audit trail* because someone could audit your project decisions or pathway.

The concept of *triangulation* also has relevance to a credible project. Related to a specific phenomenon, triangulation involves gaining two or more kinds of data, for example, gaining both interview and observation data. An example would be asking children questions about healthy meal choices as well as observing their food choices at a school cafeteria. Using more than one method to obtain a similar result improves the strength of the data (Leedy & Omrod, 2013).

Describe the Procedure/Protocol for Data Collection

After naming and describing the data-collection tools, you need to indicate a protocol for how the tools will be used in your project. This section of your proposal involves trustworthy implementation of the protocol for data collection. It is almost a "cookbook"-type approach that someone could replicate. The protocol addresses the what, how, and when questions. For a survey of students, the brief protocol could include the following: *Senior-level students will be given the survey and an informed-consent form at the end of a specified class early in the spring semester. The purpose of the survey will be broadly described to the students, and they will be asked to complete the survey and then return it at that time. Students will not receive points for completing the survey and there will be no consequences for choosing not to participate in the survey.* In addition, the protocol addresses the specific number of times the tools will be administered, such as a pretest to collect baseline data and a posttest to gain a repeated measure.

Or, in another example, if your project involves a patient room safety observations checklist, you would have already noted your plan to use a tool with good reliability and validity (or gained content-expert review of a checklist developed from review of the literature). Additional plans to be described in the proposal include approaches such as the following: *Specified observation data from the "safety checklist" will be gained from 10 occupied rooms each weekend over a period of 3 weeks. The safety checklist will be completed by the project director.* As can be noted, the protocol further defines the observations including the who, what, and when of the observations. Another investigator might, for example, want to complete a project that included observations over weekdays to see whether similarities or differences existed.

Similar protocols are needed to plan for interviews or when handing out written surveys. Protocols need to provide enough direction that others could critique a protocol's strengths and weaknesses or replicate the protocol in a similar setting.

Pilot Testing of Tools and Methods

As you make plans for consistent, reliable data collection, pretesting or piloting your tools and procedures can help identify any potential problems. Before you hand your survey to 50 people, you want to make sure the setting, procedures, and the survey itself will make them comfortable in responding.

It is important to pilot test, or pretest, your survey form. You want to make sure your project participants understand the survey questions you are sharing and how to honestly respond. For example, if you are using a qualitative survey and ask, "Could you share an experience about a safety issue?" some respondents might respond yes and then move on. This phrasing, if not caught in a pilot test, would make you miss the rich data you were seeking. Piloting would remind you to rephrase this, changing the instruction to something like "Please share an experience involving a safety issue." Another consideration to keep in mind: If you ask about certain benefits to an item such as a new staffing plan and all respondents answer "none," you are also missing data. It is often useful to add a survey question like "What else would you like to say about this topic?" or "What other thoughts do you have on this topic?"

How many people should you include in the pilot? Although no numbers are given, at least three people would give you a small range of experiences to get diverse feedback/perspectives. In addition to piloting surveys, you should also pilot observation checklists or document review forms so that others who might use these can help clarify any fuzzy points prior to data collection (Leedy & Omord, 2013). Quick tips for planning data collection are noted in Box 12.2.

BOX 12.2

Quick Tips for Data Collection

You should use good tools and be systematic in using them. Points to consider:

- Describe instruments and procedures (qualitative, quantitative, or mixed) that will be used to gain data or assess the effectiveness of an implementation.

(continued)

> **BOX 12.2** *(continued)*
>
> • Report efforts to validate and test reliability of assessment instruments.
> • Describe the protocol for collecting the data.
> • Include any needed methods for training others in data collection and piloting the data-collection plan.

● ● ●

OTHER CONSIDERATIONS

Potential challenges exist in data collection. Address each of the following as part of your methods section to promote an efficient and effective project (Krathwohl & Smith, 2005).

The Setting

Name your setting for data collection. If you plan to have students complete surveys electronically during class, you have to ensure that on a particular day, time, and place, students would bring or have access to their electronic devices for data entry. Additional consideration in describing the setting even include noting whether you plan to bring snacks for all students to the classroom. Further evaluating sites for access and appropriateness of the project and data collection are described as part of project feasibility in Chapter 10.

Data Organization

As data are collected, you will need plans that include logging the data. For example, if 50 surveys, all having 20 questions, are completed via paper and pencil, the stack of 50 surveys will not be useful to you. If you are not using an electronic survey format, your proposal should indicate who will transcribe data and what type of timeline will be used for the transcription. In many cases, this will include first transcribing to a program such as Excel, so that you can review data for completeness and any patterns in responses. Then, in many cases, you will have to transfer the data to a software program such as SPSS Statistics for computing further analyses.

Storing Data

Also address where you will store the collected data. It is especially important to note plans to store your data in a secure place, typically, a locked file that others cannot access. This is required if you ensure confidentiality of the data. Further issues in ensuring data confidentiality are addressed in Chapter 14.

Data-Collection Timeline

Your proposal needs a timeline to guide and promote consistency in data collection and progress (Krathwohl & Smith, 2005). This timeline includes attention to the who, what, and when of data collection. For example, if you are seeking to survey graduating student nurses on their readiness to practice in a culture of safety, your survey would need to be administered while they were still finishing courses. An error in timelines (or not planning far enough ahead for human subjects) could miss the data-collection point or postpone it by a full semester or even a year. Have a specific timeline in mind that determines when is the best time to collect your data.

Technology and Data Collection

There are both benefits and challenges in using technology in data collection. Benefits include rapid access to surveys for participants and easy access to collected data for the project director. Challenges include ensuring that all participants have easy access to the technologies needed (at the right time and place) and that you can gain reasonable access to an online program for moving the survey online (Leedy & Omrod, 2013).

Additional considerations for technology include its value in gaining secondary data from databases already in existence such as electronic health records (EHRs) and the National Database of Nursing Quality Indicators (NDNQI). The value of technology is also noted for organizing and analyzing data. This includes technologies such as spreadsheets for organizing, coding, and sorting simple qualitative data or for simple descriptive and basic quantitative data calculations.

● ● ●

FURTHER CHALLENGES

Instrument Development

In general, it is best to avoid developing your own instrument for a clinical project, especially if a well-developed instrument already exists. Extensive time and work are involved in instrument development, including recommended graduate coursework. If there is need for a simple survey and none exist in your project area of interest, generating questions supported in the literature or from experience can be a starting point. There are then benefits in gaining review by expert raters, a type of content validity, for supporting that the questions to be asked accurately reflect the topic you are trying to learn more about.

Project Internal Validity

Recall from previous coursework that internal validity, or ensuring the project results are due to your intervention, is critical in making the case for your findings. You have to help ensure that alternate explanations are not the cause of your outcomes. Controlling variables helps to keep the project as tight as possible to increase confidence in your findings. At minimum, be prepared to discuss variables that may influence your findings. Further reading and consultation with your mentor are needed to address this concept.

Also learn from the experience of doctor of nursing practice (DNP) students who have preceded you in completing project proposals. Their advice is presented in the following box.

● ● ●

ADVICE FROM DNP STUDENTS

Data-Collection Strategies
Be clear in relating data-collection plans
- It's not "I will collect data" but a detailed description of each point: the who will, when will, and where will data be collected.

Keep your study analysis in mind
- I am learning more about types of data (nominal, ordinal, interval, and ratio) and that is important because you can only use them in a certain way. That makes a lot of difference in how you set up a tool to gather the information and what you can do with it.

SUMMARY

This chapter has addressed strategies for your clinical project proposal that promote confidence in the tools used and help to ensure that the resultant findings are reliable and valid. Being clear in describing project tools and protocols is key.

NEXT CHAPTER UP

After collecting data, you move to analyzing and reporting your data. Strategies for analyzing qualitative data and quantitative data are shared. An important focus will be on extending your descriptive data report to include analysis.

LEARNING ACTIVITIES

To-Do List

1. Summarize your plan for data collection, including any tools you plan to use and your protocol/procedure, in a one- to two-page abstract-type format.
2. Discuss the strengths and weaknesses of your plan with your mentor. This synthesis of your ideas provides an easy communication tool for your team members.

REFERENCES

Bonnel, D. (2011). *Physical therapist assistant students' attitudes towards electronic health records* (Unpublished senior project). Washburn University, Topeka, KS.

Krathwohl, D., & Smith, N. (2005). *How to prepare a dissertation proposal: Suggestions for students in education and the social and behavioral sciences.* Syracuse, NY: Syracuse University Press.

Leedy, P., & Omrod, J. (2013). *Practical research: Planning and design* (10th ed.). Boston, MA: Pearson.

Nelson, J., & Watson, J. (2011). *Measuring caring: International research on caritas as healing.* New York, NY: Springer Publishing.

Polit, D., & Beck, C. T. (2012). *Nursing research generating and assessing evidence for nursing practice* (9th ed.). Baltimore, MD: Lippincott Williams & Wilkins.

Walker, S., Sechrist, K., & Pender, N. (1987). The health-promoting lifestyle profile: Development and psychometric characteristics. *Nursing Research, 36*(2), 76–81.

2.1

Y FORM: OPINIONS ABOUT ELECTRONIC HEALTH RECORDS

Instructions: Please circle your response to each of the following items.

1. Learning skills for using an electronic health record (EHR) are important in my health care professions education.

Strongly disagree	Disagree	Agree	Strongly agree

I plan to use EHRs in the following ways (items 2–6):

2. Logging patient care

Strongly disagree	Disagree	Agree	Strongly agree

3. Patient progress notes

Strongly disagree	Disagree	Agree	Strongly agree

4. Patient billing purposes

Strongly disagree	Disagree	Agree	Strongly agree

5. Accessing information from other disciplines to support patient care

Strongly disagree	Disagree	Agree	Strongly agree

6. I do not plan to use EHRs in my practice.

Strongly disagree	Disagree	Agree	Strongly agree

The benefits I see to using EHRs include (items 7–9):

7. Help make my documentation more complete

Strongly disagree	Disagree	Agree	Strongly agree

8. Help me minimize errors

Strongly disagree	Disagree	Agree	Strongly agree

9. Help me increase my efficiency

Strongly disagree	Disagree	Agree	Strongly agree

10. I am adequately proficient in EHR skills.

Strongly disagree	Disagree	Agree	Strongly agree

Instructions: Please write in your written response to the following items:

11. The challenges or problems I see to using EHRs include . . .

12. Where/when did you receive the most information about using EHRs in your practice?

Source: Adapted from Bonnel (2011).

Writing Your Proposal: Adding the Detail for Proposal Completion

13

Writing the Data-Analysis Plans for Advanced Clinical Projects

Reflective Questions

In Chapter 12, you considered various issues related to collecting valid and reliable data for your proposal plans. In this chapter, you will consider how best to propose plans for analyzing your data. The following reflective questions organize learning for this chapter. With which of the following are you most comfortable?

- Beginning to plan data organizing, analyzing, and reporting?
- Considering strategies and rationale for varied data-analysis approaches?
- Writing the analysis plan, including addressing benefits/challenges of organizing full analysis plans in the proposal?

This chapter focuses on your proposal plans for organizing/reporting and analyzing the data you collect. Strategies for analyzing subject characteristics, qualitative data, and quantitative data are shared. An important focus will be writing plans that focus on analyzing, rather than merely listing, the data obtained. As you write your proposal, this chapter also guides you in thinking it through or anticipating what your final report might look like.

• • •

DATA PLANNING

Advanced clinical projects consist of data, whether those data are newly generated data, synthesized from existing data, or evaluation data related to evidence being tested. Plans for organizing, analyzing, and reporting those data are important in the proposal plan. As it sounds, organizing the data involves organizing or describing the data that were collected. Analysis involves a detailed examination that helps you and others better understand or make sense of the data. Too often the plan for data analysis is left out or is just a mere suggestion. Reporting data involves communicating the analysis. This plan is needed at the initial proposal stage or you are likely to end up with problems or a gap in what you wanted to convey.

In planning for the organizing, analyzing, and reporting components of your proposal, remember that this plan is not an afterthought, but a key component of the project purpose (refer back to the methods point on the project triangle). To accomplish this, the project plan will need to include how the collected data will initially be retrieved and organized. This prospective approach also helps ensure that needed data are being collected before it is time for the analysis.

For example, if your project involves surveying 30 people, each responding to 10 items, you will want to know their individual responses to items as well as the group's collective responses to items. This allows you to look for patterns, both in individual responses across items as well as the full group response across items. An easy way to gain this big picture of the data is to review the data in an Excel spreadsheet. Creating a "person by item" table allows both review of each individual's responses to survey items, seeking any patterns, as well as opportunity to review summative average responses to each item. Paying "prospective" attention to data analysis is the focus of this chapter.

• • •

ANALYZING DATA

Although organizing data is an important first step, it is essentially just a listing of the data, or what was attained. Without showing how the data have been reviewed/considered through meaningful analysis, the numbers just become a long laundry list (i.e., long lists of community health data are not very useful unless they are organized into meaningful categories for comparisons). Analysis involves "meaning-making" of the data. For example, you may report the following total scores on a knowledge posttest given to community members about smoking cessation: 75, 34, 89, 52, and 61. However, those scores are meaningless unless accompanied by analysis criteria and interpretation. So what might have looked like a good, high score of 89 suddenly looks dismal when analysis guidelines indicate a total of 150 points is the possible high score and the higher the score the better.

* * *

YOUR PROPOSAL: OVERVIEW OF PLANNING FOR DATA ANALYSIS

Once your purpose statement, methods, and outcomes are identified, your detailed methods section then provides direction for your analysis plans. The goal is to organize and plan an analysis that ties to the clinical questions addressed. Thinking through your project analysis requires anticipating what your final report might look like.

Literally every project will require some type of data analysis. For any clinical project that organizes data or evidence already available, or collects new data for evaluation of a protocol or to explore new topical areas, some type of data analysis is required. There are often multiple options for completing data analysis. For example, all projects will have descriptive statistics that describe sample characteristics. Depending on the project purpose/question and methods, further data gained from this sample may then be presented as descriptive analysis or inferential analysis. Understanding the background of these approaches and why they are important is key. The characteristics of your sample and qualitative-analysis and quantitative-analysis approaches are further described in the following sections.

Your Proposal: Plan for Descriptive Data and Sample Characteristics

Your proposal analysis plan will include an initial report of descriptive data. In almost all cases, this will include a descriptive analysis of the data collected (the interviews/surveys/observations/records reviewed). This means you will have to think ahead about how descriptive data will be shared. If you are interviewing clinicians, the characteristics you want to describe about them will have to match any demographic surveys you provide them (so you will make sure you have the correct questions on your survey to match with what you want to say about the sample). For example, if surveying clinicians, you will often want to know about their background or who they are. What characteristics about them are important to your clinical project? How many participated and what did they "look" like (i.e., How old are they? How long have they practiced? What are their specialties?)?

While you are considering the characteristics you want to describe, it also makes sense to think ahead about how you will report this information. Think ahead about the tables you will want to share after the data are collected. Proposal completion involves detailing even to the point of building blank tables for description, including charts/boxes that hold a place for descriptive findings in your final report.

Your Proposal: Plan for Sharing Qualitative Results

If you have used a data-collection approach, such as a survey asking open-ended questions about your topic, you will have to make plans for qualitative data analysis. Your analysis plans will include review of responses to these open-ended questions to seek common themes. Themes provide a way of conveying what has been learned from long lists of word responses. It is a way to interpret and make data meaningful. In essence, the goal is to learn how a topic is perceived by subjects or written about in documents (Berg, 2008).

Content analysis provides a way to gain themes from the qualitative data. In some ways it serves as a funnel, first seeking broad pictures from the data and then seeking additional patterns. It can provide a way to identify, organize, index, and retrieve data. It is asking questions of the data that relate back to the study purpose. Content analysis focuses on themes, messages, or key points in the data. Content analysis begins with:

- *Reviewing raw data*: listing and considering
- *Organizing*: creating files
- *Examining/perusing*: getting an overview, listing preliminary thoughts
- *Classifying*: putting data into categories/themes
- *Synthesizing*: generate tables, diagrams, hypothesize relationships

A theme is considered a simple phrase that captures an idea or concept. Some projects will use a priori coding to seek themes. This means that selected categories are named before the data are reviewed. The categories are then used in reviewing and seeing whether they are found in the data. For example, do the data responses correspond to a set criteria, such as supportive or nonsupportive, of a new practice policy? Another approach uses "open" coding. With open coding, themes emerge as common responses are heard multiple times. For example, in a qualitative survey of new charge nurses, data might reflect common concerns, or themes, about learning how to staff a unit or engage the team. Themes sometimes emerge as you ask what surprises me about these results.

Content Analysis Example

Referring to the electronic health record (EHR) survey example, supplied in the last chapter (see Appendix 12.1), content analysis was used for open-ended question responses (the last two survey items). For example, in completing content analysis of one specific open-ended survey question "The challenges or problems I see to using EHRs include . . .," from the 22 phrases received, the following themes were identified: issues for training, problems with access, concerns about losing data, and privacy issues. Each theme would then be further described and specific examples for each category provided.

Your Proposal: Plan for Sharing Descriptive Quantitative Results

Quantitative data analysis provides a way of summarizing your data through numbers. If quantitative data will be gained, planning choices for analysis include considering whether descriptive statistics only will be appropriate, or will descriptive statistics plus inferential statistics best convey the data findings? In any of the analyses chosen, the goal is to address the project questions. For example, in planning to evaluate staff satisfaction with a specific staff development program, all responses to a specific survey item (rating 1–4 high) could be summarized according to range, mean, and standard deviation. In addition, the item scores can be averaged for a specific group and their scores reported in a similar fashion. If there is intent to compare satisfaction ratings between new staff and experienced staff, then an inferential statistic, such as the t-test, would be used to compare these two groups' mean satisfaction score (a type of inferential statistic). The analysis plan will relate back to the project triangle, with a focus on the methods, including sampling plan and type of data collected (as further described in the following text).

Descriptive quantitative components are a type of counting used to create a numerical picture of the data. They can include a count of contextual elements and might use, for example, tally sheets or frequency counts. These can be created by hand, but, as noted, technology makes generating these counts fairly easy. Appendices 13.1 and 13.2 provide examples of tables using frequency counts.

Your Proposal: Inferential Quantitative Data-Analysis Plans

If you are using inferential statistics, then you analyze your data to see whether there are unique findings (showing statistical significance) or whether your findings were more probably related to chance. Inferential statistics involve meeting assumptions for inferential statistics (e.g., large sample size, usually noted to be greater than 30 to approximate a normal curve that the statistics are based on). In addition, to know you are choosing the correct inferential tests, you will need to describe the level of data in your data collection. Data-analysis tests are guided by the level of data being analyzed:

- *Nominal*: This type of data can be put in unique categories in which the answer is 1 of 2 options. These include, for example, responses to questions that ask about categories like yes/no or black/white. Modes will be reported descriptively; then further analysis with nonparametric tests, such as the chi-square test, can be used for category comparisons.
- *Ordinal*: This type of data can be ordered, such as data from "good, better, best" type surveys. These data will typically be described/reported with medians/ranges; then further analysis can be used with nonparametric tests like the Wilcoxon signed ranks test.
- *Interval/ratio*: This type of data can be used mathematically, such as numerical scores on a knowledge test. Mean/averages and standard deviations are reported descriptively; then further analysis is done with parametric statistics, such as *t*-tests, analysis of variance (ANOVA), or other tests, depending on the project purpose.

Describe the Inferential Statistics to Be Used

Once you identify the level of data, return to your handy statistics text to confirm you are planning the right test for your type of data (consulting with your mentor is also a good idea). For instance, in a continuing-education program example, it might be appropriate to compare mean program satisfaction scores between new staff and experienced staff using an independent *t*-test.

A good guide for those new to advanced clinical project data-analysis plans is to select only the core variables for simple inferential testing. Again, indicate any plans to complete simple inferential tests as part of the project proposal. As you work on this section of your proposal, you will want additional readings/references to support your plans. If you are new to this process, a useful reference such as *Statistics for People Who (Think They) Hate Statistics* (Salkind, 2011) can be helpful. More complex approaches to analysis can be considered with your mentor.

• • •

MAKING A PLAN FOR REPORTING THE DATA ANALYSIS: VISUAL PRESENTATION

Plan to Organize Results

Even though you have no data at the proposal stage, making plans to organize your descriptive data and data analyses provides a "step up" when it is time for the analysis phase of your project. Consider the value of a large three-ring binder or its electronic equivalent. If your project will end with the traditional five scholarly sections, put five dividers in this binder at the beginning of project implementation as a reminder of, or placeholder for the final sections. This basically requires visualizing, at the proposal stage, the project as processed and completed. In preparation for the data you will soon acquire, data-analysis plans can even include the blank table formats. Although this advice is easy to ignore, addressing this advice will pay dividends in saved time and frustration later.

As you plan to communicate your final project results, you will want to visually showcase these in your final project paper. Generate plans for tables or charts that can be used to document descriptive characteristics of project subjects as well as further data analyses from surveys or other tools. Tables and charts help organize data that are too complex to just convey through paragraph form. Those who will read your final project paper will often find it easiest to skim your tables and charts to quickly identify findings. Creating these placeholders now for future data also provides you time to make sure you are collecting the correct data to address your purpose statement. Making this plan now may even make it easier to complete the write-up of these sections as you work with these established tables (Box 13.1).

BOX 13.1

Writing the Data-Analysis Plan

The following example provides a sample analysis plan for a hypothetical EHRs project. The project purpose is to identify perceptions of clinical students on readiness to use EHRs in their employment settings postgraduation. Using the EHR survey example, supplied in Appendix 12.1, the following paragraph provides a brief summary evaluation plan, for the 10-item quantitative survey and two-item qualitative questions.

(continued)

BOX 13.1 *(continued)*

Data analysis will be completed with basic descriptive statistics used to describe the 10 structured-response items. An Excel spreadsheet of each participant's responses will be shared (see Appendices 13.1 and 13.2). This will allow for review of the numeric data for patterns. A frequency-count table will be constructed to further analyze subject responses with appropriate histograms generated. Qualitative responses to the two open-ended items will be typed verbatim into a word-processing program. Content analysis seeking themes will be completed by the researcher and a second health professional.

• • •

QUICK TIPS

Sometimes it is easiest to start by sharing the descriptive data and then summarizing how these data answer the project question(s). At minimum include:

- *Subject demographics*: Descriptive statistics are used for sharing demographic data. Share your plans for completing tables or bullets with frequencies and ranges of responses for each demographic item.
- *Closed-ended (limited response) items*: Descriptive statistics are used for conveying responses to survey items that are closed-ended. Share plans for completing tables or bullets with frequencies and central tendency measures for each item on a survey or checklist (as well as total scores if using a validated tool).
- *Open-ended (descriptive response) items*: Common themes are gained from open-ended survey items and content analysis. Plan to share common themes identified from these items, for example, in bullet-list form or a summary table.

• • •

PLANNING AHEAD FOR PROJECT COMPLETION: DISCUSSION/IMPLICATIONS

After implementing your proposal and completing your project data analysis, you will establish conclusions and recommendations. These will be based on the synthesis of evidence from your project and related to your project purpose. These sections will help you address the "so what?" of findings from the project.

Even in the planning phase it is important to consider potential project implications. Often, implications will be considered, at minimum, in terms of further implications for practice, education, and research. For example, in the EHR project example in this chapter, the following implications might emerge for the discussion section of a final report.

- *For practice*: It is important for academic and practice settings to work together in preparing students for future clinical work with EHRs.
- *For education*: Further education is recommended across classroom and clinical settings.
- *For further research*: Further study of the best ways to learn and use EHRs is recommended.

After project implementation your results and discussion/implications sections will be components of your final project report. Plan to create a scholarly document to be presented and defended to your community of interest as well as other stakeholders, academic communities, and interested parties.

As you move forward in your work, consider the experiences of doctor of nursing practice (DNP) students who have already completed project proposals. Their advice is presented in the following box.

ADVICE FROM DNP STUDENTS

Data-Analysis Strategies

Know analysis plans prior to collecting data
- I learned that it is imperative to think about and have an idea of the type of data you will obtain, how you will utilize it, and why you choose the method of analysis you did.
- Know ahead of time what statistics you will use. This serves as a check and helps make sure you are gaining the right data.

Know levels of data
- Walk away understanding nominal, ordinal, interval, and ratio data. I never understood the terms before.

Think about tools available to you
- Learn about programs, like Excel, that you can use to manage data.

(continued)

• • •

ADVICE FROM DNP STUDENTS ON DATA ANALYSIS STRATEGIES
(continued)

Appreciate the value of showing or providing visuals of the data
* Create blank tables as part of the proposal. Become savvy in use of tables and graphs for data visualization.

Don't write about an analysis that will not apply
* The most challenging parts for me are trying to determine the data analysis that will be utilized for my project and creating tables before you even have the data.

Use your previous coursework on research and epidemiology
* Pull out the "practical/applied stats" book and review statistics that you will need for your project.

SUMMARY

Planning for data collection and analysis in your project go hand in hand. Proactive planning helps avoid the problem of gaining too much, not enough, or the wrong data. This chapter provided direction for thinking ahead to final components of the project, including organizing and analyzing the data you collect. You will want to make credible plans for data analysis so that all can clearly understand your project results.

NEXT CHAPTER UP

Being ethical and accountable in your project work is a key component of clinical scholarship. Key ethical issues for project proposals will be addressed.

LEARNING ACTIVITIES

To-Do List

Review your data-analysis plans and address the following questions.

1. What is your level of data?
2. What are your analysis plans?

3. How do your plans flow from the purpose statement?
4. How do your analysis plans set the stage for displaying and discussing your results?
5. Does your mentor agree with your analysis?

REFERENCES

Berg, B. (2008) *Qualitative research methods for the social sciences* (7th ed.). Boston, MA: Pearson.

Salkind, N. (2011). *Statistics for people who (think they) hate statistics*. Thousand Oaks, CA: Sage.

APPENDIX 13.1

SAMPLE FREQUENCY COUNT: OPINIONS ABOUT ELECTRONIC HEALTH RECORDS[a]

ITEMS	SD	D	A	SA	COUNT TOTAL
1.	1	0	12	9	22
2.	1	0	15	6	22
3.	0	0	13	9	22
4.	1	0	10	11	22
5.	0	1	11	10	22
6.	13	8	1	0	22
7.	0	0	14	8	22
8.	1	0	14	7	22
9.	1	0	11	10	22
10.	13	6	3	0	22

SD = strongly disagree; A = agree; D = disagree; SA = strongly agree.

[a]Review the sample survey form, Opinions About Electronic Health Records, provided in Appendix 12.1. This example provides data using that tool. The number of respondents, for each item option from the sample survey, is $N = 22$. Under each of the response categories, the number of total respondents answering in that category is provided.

DESCRIPTIVE RESULTS: OPINIONS ABOUT ELECTRONIC HEALTH RECORDS[a]

ITEMS	1	2	3	4	5	6	7	8	9	10
Subject 1	3	3	3	2	3	2	3	3	2	2
2	3	3	3	4	1	3	3	3	3	2
3	3	3	3	3	3	1	4	4	4	1
4	3	3	3	3	3	1	3	3	3	2
5	3	3	3	3	3	2	3	3	3	1
6	4	4	4	4	4	2	3	3	3	2
7	4	4	3	3	4	2	3	3	4	2
8	3	3	3	3	3	2	3	3	3	2
9	4	3	4	4	3	2	4	4	4	2
10	4	3	3	3	4	2	3	3	3	3
11	3	3	3	3	3	2	3	3	3	1
12	4	4	4	4	4	1	4	4	4	2
13	3	3	3	3	3	2	3	3	3	1
14	4	3	4	4	4	1	4	4	4	2
15	2	3	3	3	4	2	3	2	4	1
16	4	3	3	4	3	2	3	4	4	2
17	3	4	4	4	4	1	4	3	4	3
18	3	3	3	3	3	1	3	3	3	2
19	3	4	4	4	4	1	4	3	3	3
20	3	3	4	4	3	2	3	4	4	2
21	4	4	4	4	4	1	4	4	4	2
22	3	3	4	4	4	2	3	3	3	1
Average										
	3.30	3.27	3.41	3.45	3.36	1.68	3.31	3.27	3.41	1.86
Standard Deviation										
	0.57	0.46	0.50	0.60	0.73	0.57	0.48	0.55	0.59	0.64
Mode										
	3	3	3	4	3	2	3	3	3	2
Median										
	3	3	3	3.5	3	2	3	3	3	2

[a]Again, review the survey form, Opinions About Electronic Health Records, provided in Appendix 12.1. This table provides basic descriptive data showing how each of the 22 respondents marked each survey item. Setting up a table such as this allows you to look for patterns.

14

...

Keeping Clinical Projects
Ethical and Dependable

Reflective Questions

You've spent a lot of time working on your project. You've reviewed and organized the literature, honed the purpose statement, and determined what methods and data analysis you'll use. One issue that impacts all of these activities, but has not yet been addressed, is how to do all of this in an ethical manner. The following reflective questions organize learning for this chapter. With which of the following are you most comfortable?

- How do professional competencies and standards extend to clinical projects?
- Why is discussion of ethical issues important in clinical projects?
- What do these concepts mean in planning and writing a proposal?

● ● ●

PROFESSIONALISM AND PROFESSIONAL STANDARDS

Because in the last chapter you just read about analyzing your data, you may feel like you are about done with your clinical project proposal. However, this is a case in which some of the most important content has been saved for last. Your project will not receive the desired recognition or acceptance if it has not been conducted with the utmost integrity, and so you need to be sure that all ethical aspects of the project have been identified and addressed.

All nurses are required to adhere to nursing's professional values and standards. Standards have been established by a number of professional nursing organizations to guide the implementation of those values. The American Nurses Association's (ANA) *Scope and Standards of Practice* (2010) is one such document. When you move into scholarly work with your clinical project, then additional standards and competencies apply. For example, when writing a formal paper such as the proposal, a specific writing style is identified and applied. In nursing, that is often the American Psychological Association's (APA; 2010) writing style, although other styles are also used. Some ethical standards and competencies extend beyond nursing to interprofessional teamwork. For example, the book *Core Competencies for Interprofessional Collaborative Practice* (Interprofessional Education Collaborative Expert Panel, 2011) has been developed and includes competency domains for values and ethics for interprofessional practice, roles and responsibilities, interprofessional communication, and teams and teamwork. Also, whenever you participate in conducting research on human subjects, the *Federal Policy for the Protection of Human Subjects* (2010) details pertinent guidelines. Using these documents can be key to completing successful professional projects.

• • •

KEY ETHICAL STANDARDS

Give Credit Where Credit Is Due

Recognizing and acknowledging the work of others is a fundamental element of scholarly writing. Whenever you use someone else's exact words, or even someone else's ideas paraphrased in your own words, you must give that person credit. Failure to recognize ideas and words that belong to someone else as his or her work, and not yours, constitutes plagiarism. Although this may seem like a simple concept, it can be deceptive. The easiest case is when you are the author of a paper (the clinical project proposal, or any paper on which you are acknowledged as the author) and you include ideas that are your own thoughts that are written in your own words, and which you have never published before, then you can simply write them down and move on.

A slightly more complicated case is when you are writing your own thoughts or words, which you have previously published. In this case, and because of copyright laws, you must reference your previous thoughts or words, even though they all came from you. The failure to reference your own previous work is called *self-plagiarism.*

A much clearer example of plagiarism is when you use or refer to someone else's ideas or words and fail to give that person credit. Credit is given by correctly referencing the source of the words or ideas, so that readers can go to that source and see the original words or ideas themselves. This practice of referencing has very important implications for your proposal.

- When you use someone else's exact words, you must insert quotation marks or italicize their words and provide the source in which those exact words can be found.
- When you use someone else's ideas, and even if you paraphrase the ideas using your own words to describe the other person's ideas, then you must also provide the source in which that exact idea can be found.
- Provide the source in which those words and/or ideas that you are referencing can be found exactly as prescribed by the writing style you are using.

Permission to Use Instruments

Although any number of research instruments are available for use in the public domain and may therefore be used by anyone (with appropriate referencing, of course), there are a number of instruments that do not fall into that category. Permission is required to use instruments that are unpublished and developed by someone else, as well as instruments that have been copyrighted. In both cases, you must receive formal permission to use the instruments, and that written permission must be (a) referenced in the proposal narrative and (b) provided in the appendices.

Conflict of Interest

Conflict of interest refers to when researchers do not maintain unbiased objectivity because they have something at stake or competing interests (most often, but not always, something to gain) that include some aspect(s) of the research they have what is referred to as a conflict of interest (Steneck, 2007). Potential financial gain is frequently the first and only example of a conflict of interest that can be identified. Conflicts of interest may also include competing responsibilities or benefits of either a personal or professional nature. A clear example of conflict of interest is a company conducting research on its own product and concluding, contrary to objective analysis of the data, that it is excellent and should be widely used. Another example is when drug representatives conduct a presentation or provide gifts or meals that encourage use of their products over a competitor's, when their competitor has no chance to respond on behalf of his or her own products. A more subtle example might be a student who participates in a project with a boss or admired colleague, in which case objectivity might be lost to the advantage of the boss or colleague. Conflicts, when they exist, do not necessarily mean that the project cannot be completed. Rather, a completely honest and transparent process that identifies the conflict(s) and applies mechanisms by which objectivity can be maintained and monitored must be implemented and documented.

Human Subjects

The most comprehensive standards in any clinical project are those regarding the use of human subjects in projects and/or research (there are also comprehensive standards for projects that include the use of animals, although that is far less common in nursing and so is not addressed in this book). Your own research cannot be started until these standards are met and you have written approval to begin. All researchers are expected to uphold the ethical principles of autonomy, justice, and beneficence (Steneck, 2007) through the self-regulation of their respective professions. That self-regulation is augmented by federal government legislation, which was formalized in 1974 when the Department of Health, Education and Welfare (HEW) codified the procedures of research under Title 45 of the Code of Federal Regulations, part 46 (45 CFR 46). In 1991 most federal agencies affiliated with human research adopted common regulation for human subject protections as 45 CFR 46, subpart A, which is commonly referred to as the *Common Rule* (*Federal Policy for the Protection of Human Subjects*, 2010).

Institutional review boards (IRBs) are established to implement and monitor the principles of research promulgated in the Common Rule at all institutions receiving federal dollars. Some proposals may be deemed exempt or expedited because they are very low risk for human subjects. It may even be determined that some clinical projects are not classified as research per se and therefore not subject to the Common Rule. Such decisions and classifications are the IRB's purview and not determined by the investigators themselves. Informed consent is one of the most complex features of the Common Rule and is closely monitored by IRBs, as it is a primary mechanism by which the ethical principles of autonomy, justice, and beneficence are upheld. For example, if your project involves research components, you must inform potential participants of

- The research background, purpose, and procedures
- Why they have been asked to participate
- Their right to not participate, without any negative repercussions
- Their right to withdraw from the study at any time without negative repercussions

- Their right to ask questions about participation
- Their right to voluntarily consent to participation without coercion
- Their right to know the benefits of participating, as well as any risks or inconveniences
- Their right to confidentiality
- Access to the researcher's contact information in case they have questions or are injured

With this information, and being as fully informed as possible, potential participants are able to make autonomous decisions about their willingness to participate in a project or not.

In addition to protecting the autonomy of all potential research participants, IRBs work to protect vulnerable populations whose autonomy may be limited. The Common Rule has in place additional protections for certain groups, such as pregnant women, human fetuses, neonates, children, and prisoners, who may be asked to participate in research studies. Many social determinants of health (environmental conditions in which people are born and/or live that affect their health and quality of life), such as exposure to crime and violence, language/literacy, and socioeconomic conditions (Healthy People 2020, 2016) may also affect potential research participants' ability to exercise full autonomy in choosing to participate in research or not. All project proposals must demonstrate your thorough analysis and plan for protecting all potential participants, especially those who, for whatever reason, may be considered vulnerable in their ability to make autonomous decisions.

If your project will require a consent form, and many projects will, several organizations provide consent-form templates for project directors. Go to your own institution's website and see whether you can find an example (Box 14.1). If you do not find a template at your own organization, or if you want to compare templates, an example is provided on the University of Missouri–Kansas City's website: (www.umkc.edu/umkc-search/?cx=008281657408603500330%3Avpif2cmpa14& cof=FORID%3A10&ie=UTF-8&q=sample%20consent%20forms).

The implications of the Common Rule are far reaching for all students and researchers conducting clinical projects with human subjects. The good news is that you only need to know that virtually all projects or research involving human subjects must be submitted to, reviewed by, and approved in writing by the IRB before it is implemented. But this IRB review process takes time, and so you need to account for that in your projected project timeline. Also, although the Common Rule provides the guidelines, each institution has its own specific policies and procedures on how the Common Rule is implemented, and so it is your responsibility to know the policies and procedures for your own institution. Keep in mind, too, that if you are associated with multiple institutions and/or will conduct the project at multiple sites, all of those sites/institutions must review the proposal and provide written approval. No aspect of the project may be started until the proposal has been reviewed and you have received written approval to proceed from the IRB.

Data Integrity

You are nearing completion of your project proposal, and you already have a wealth of time and effort invested. It is imperative that you take the time and steps necessary now to ensure the dependability of the data when you are done because, without that, your reputation and the impact of your hard work will not be respected by the scientific community and practicing nurses.

BOX 14.1

Agency Website

Visit the website(s) of your institution(s) to see what policies and procedures exist with relevance to your project proposal. Keep in mind that if you hold multiple roles (such as student and employee), or if you will use multiple project sites, you must comply with the regulations of all involved institutions.

You have already anticipated and addressed several threats to dependable and reliable, or trustworthy and transferable, data during the design and data-collection procedures of your project. For example, you chose reliable instruments, and/or you decided to use triangulation approaches. Now you must also ensure the integrity of the data through ongoing, accurate, confidential, and dependable record keeping. This process is often facilitated by keeping an ongoing log of your daily activities and decisions, as captured in an audit trail. Also be sure to check the policies and procedures at you own institution(s) to confirm how long you must keep and maintain your research data and files.

• • •

FINAL STEPS

There are lots of ethical aspects to research and other scholarly work. The best advice is to be well informed on the ethical issues and to address them up front, during the proposal phase of your clinical project. Remember to consult with project mentors on any questions. This is not an area where it is best to "ask for forgiveness afterward," so be proactive and transparent in your preparations.

Go through the entire list of ethical aspects, be absolutely honest with yourself and your team, and address each item now.

SUMMARY

This chapter has presented issues related to conducting your project in an ethical manner. Working through the IRB process can add unexpected time to the project and may result in the addition of safeguards that you had not previously considered, but the additional effort in respecting not only the integrity of your work, but also the integrity of any research participants who may be a part of your work, is an essential element of the scientific process.

WEBSITES FOR FURTHER REVIEW

Further examples of tools used for ethical decision making that can be applied when considering clinical projects include:

- The Critical Thinking series provides sample documents on ethics and opportunities to gain further tools relevant to your project plans. The Thinkers Guides *Ethical Reasoning* sample provides further information: www.criticalthinking.org/store/products/ethical-reasoning/169

Social determinants have a huge impact on health and related clinical projects. Read more about social determinants of health in:

- *A Framework for Educating Health Professionals to Address the Social Determinants of Health:*
www.nationalacademies.org/hmd/Reports/2016/Framework-for
-Educating-Health-Professionals-to-Address-the-Social
-Determinants-of-Health.aspx

NEXT CHAPTER UP

You now have a fairly complete proposal in hand, and you have addressed the ethical elements and ramifications of the project as well. Your next step is to edit, revise, and finalize the proposal so that it is ready for others to review. As you revise and edit, you will be laying the groundwork for your final project paper, and that will have widespread distribution, even publication, and you want everything to be accurate as well as conducive to finishing that final report/paper.

LEARNING ACTIVITIES

To-Do List

If your project will require consent forms, use your agency's template to start a draft of your consent form, being sure to include:

- The name of the study and researchers
- Why any individuals are being asked to participate
- A brief rationale for study and participation
- A brief explanation of the study purpose
  - A brief explanation of the study procedures and the nature of the participant's activities and time commitment
- The benefits (including any payment/compensation)
- Risks of participation (including fees)
  - That participation is voluntary, with no negative consequences if individuals choose not to participate, as well as alternatives to participation
- Individuals may withdraw at any time, without negative consequences
- Confidentiality
- Who to contact with questions/problems/injury
- Signature block for participant and consenter

_____

_____

_____

_____

_____

_____

_____

_____

REFERENCES

American Nurses Association. (2010). *Scope and standards of practice* (2nd ed.). Silver Spring, MD: Author.

American Psychological Association. (2010). *Publication manual of the American Psychological Association* (6th ed.). Washington, DC: Author.

Federal Policy for the Protection of Human Subjects. (2010). 45 CFR 46, subpart A. Retrieved from http://www.hhs.gov/ohrp/humansubjects/guidance/45cfr46.html

Healthy People 2020. (2016). Social determinants of health. Retrieved from https://www.healthypeople.gov/2020/topics-bjectives/topic/social-determinants-of-health

Interprofessional Education Collaborative Expert Panel. (2011). *Core competencies for interprofessional collaborative practice: Report of an expert panel.* Washington, DC: Author.

Steneck, N. H. (2007). Office of Research Integrity: Introduction to the responsible conduct of research. Retrieved from http://ori.hhs.gov/documents/rcrintro.pdf

15

...

Finalizing the Proposal as a Professional Document: Reviewing, Editing, and Revising

Reflective Questions

In Chapter 14, you reviewed considerations for proposing and conducting your project in an ethical manner. In this chapter, you will be approaching a final proposal step of editing, revising, and finalizing your proposal so that it is ready for others to review. The following reflective questions organize learning for this chapter. With which of the following are you most comfortable?

- Finalizing the proposal draft (including edits/revisions) as a professional document?
- Considering next steps in using the proposal for moving toward project completion?
- Optimizing use of self-assessment and the project team to finalize the proposal?

As you finalize your proposal you are striving to become precise in your language to make sure your readers understand clearly what you mean. As clinicians advance their education and their standing in the health care arena, professional written communication becomes even more important a tool. Project proposals have applications in many arenas and underscore the value of this professional document. Previous chapters have focused on the content to include in a proposal. This chapter finalizes planning for the professional document. It involves tailoring the writing to the professional audience. It also includes continuing the ideas/plans into the next phases of implementing the project and thinking ahead to how the project results and discussion will be conveyed.

• • •

EDITING/REVISING THE FIRST DRAFT

Clear communication is central to scholarly work. Often, people write out plans they think are perfectly clear but then realize the information is only clear to them (of course they already know what they are doing—now clarifying the wording so others understand is key). Although the initial drafts are a matter of "getting it down in writing" and making it clear to yourself, the final draft is about making written communication clear to others. This means reflecting on the current draft (what has been produced or written?) and what still needs to be done to finalize the proposal. It includes the use of precise language and maintaining consistency with terms to make sure your reader can understand and easily follow your meaning. Communication models support sending clear messages that others can interpret and respond to via feedback.

• • •

COMPLETING THE FINAL PROPOSAL

The hallmark of completing the proposal is paying attention to all of the details, including the proposal substance, structure, appendices, and writing/editing. Your table of contents can serve you well in organizing your narrative and providing good direction for you and your readers. Suggested questions to guide proposal completion are included in the following section.

• • •

QUESTIONS TO GUIDE YOU IN DETAILING THE PROPOSAL

Proposal Substance

Conveying important content that helps enhance your project proposal is key. Make sure you have addressed the following:

- Is the project purpose important in helping care for or benefit your population of interest?
- Is the proposal purpose statement clearly written and consistently re-stated throughout the proposal?

- Are the three triangle anchors—purpose, methods, and outcomes—consistent throughout the proposal?
- Have summaries been used to repeat key section ideas for reader clarity?

Proposal Structure

Writing a proposal that meets scholarly criteria for communicating with other professionals is key. Are the following proposal sections clearly identified and written in scholarly format?

- Introductory section clarifying the project problem and purpose
- Review of the literature
- Methods section

Proposal Appendices

The appendices must be complete, and referred to in the narrative. Do they include the following points?

- The data-collection tools and any needed permissions forms, if using developed tools
- Agency agreements to complete the project
- Needed human subjects approvals
- Any consent forms (approved format)

Writing/Editing

Self-editing is an early step in finalizing your proposal. The following basic guides can provide a useful starting point:

- Has the approved writing style (such as that of the American Psychological Association [APA]) been used correctly and consistently?
- Has clear wording been used?
- Have consistent tenses been used throughout?
- Have terms and abbreviations been appropriately introduced and referred to consistently throughout?
- Have headings been used to their best advantage to help outline the content and facilitate smooth flow of content? These headings link the proposal parts together, provide cues for the reader, and keep the reader moving forward.
- Has all cited work been referenced appropriately?

• • •

FURTHER WRITING TIPS

Staying clear with your message is key. Further tips for clarifying your written proposal include:

- *Avoid excessive use of abbreviations and avoid confusing abbreviations*: For example, if you are referring to mental illness as "MI," medical–surgical nurses will immediately think about myocardial infarction. Again, be sure all abbreviations are properly introduced per your respective writing-style guidelines.
- *Use appropriate terms appropriately (do not mix concepts)*: Define the terms you will be using in the initial sections of the proposal. For example, "simulation" is sometimes used to indicate standardized patients and other times to describe high-fidelity technology-supported simulation. Be clear about what you mean.
- *Stay consistent with key terms*: Do a final "search" on the main terms (and any that you have described as interchangeable) and make sure they are consistent in all sections of the proposal. Go back and see what terms you used early on and confirm consistent use throughout the proposal.
- *Use summary statements*: Summary statements can be powerful in tying parts of a proposal together.
- *Use scholarly language; be precise in methods language*: Especially for similar-sounding terms, be careful to use the right term. For example, do not mix up the terms *content validity* and *content analysis*.
- *Seek consistency in lists*: Items should include consistent phrasing. For example, if the first item uses the "ing" phrase, then all successive items on the list should be written in the same way (i.e., *caring, coupling*, and *changing*).
- *Punctuate*: Make sure that sentences are not too long and hard to follow. Can you read each sentence aloud and still breathe at the end?
- *Keep paragraph lengths appropriate*: Avoid creating a page full of sentences or a "wall of words" that is hard to follow. One strategy to avoid this is to be sure you use paragraphs of appropriate length.
- *Write using the recommended style*: Although there are a variety of writing styles and you should use whatever you have been directed to follow, APA is the style often used in nursing. The style guidelines will direct all aspects of your final written proposal. For example, APA uses the third-person format (the typical scholarly format). If first person is preferred, check first with your reviewing source/agency.
- *Read the full project draft*: This helps you gain the big picture; you can then focus on needed details (Galvan, 2013).

* * *

FINALIZING THE TIMELINE AND PROJECT BUDGET

If not previously addressed in the proposal, now is the time to consider the project timeline and budget. These are two valuable components that keep a project moving forward.

What Is the Project Timeline?

Although you have been thinking tentatively about a timeline for your project, this is the time to finalize it. As you return to your project map, consider what needs to happen when. List out each component of the proposal requiring an action and generate a best estimate of a time frame. One of the benefits of Word tables or Excel spreadsheets is that they help you stay on track and communicate your plan clearly to others.

What Is the Project Budget?

Although you have been thinking tentatively about a budget for your project proposal, now is the time to finalize this essential element. Some clinical projects will have minimal budgets that will be subsumed as part of the work contribution to a setting. Sometimes there will be costs such as preparing surveys and/or providing snacks for participants. Consider and note these items.

If the proposal is being submitted for some type of grant funding, the project budget will be large enough to require a specific budget and budget justification. Excel spreadsheets can assist in clearly documenting and justifying the budget.

* * *

NEXT STEPS FOR THE PROPOSAL

To help you keep on track for implementing and completing your project proposal, now is the time to give thought to your project completion and final analysis and write-up. This will involve attending to sections of your final project write-up, including planning for the results, discussion, and implications sections.

Planning for the Results Section

How will you describe the results you gain from data collection? Remember to build in paragraphs that convey plans for completing sections four and five: the sections for results of the project and the discussion of the findings. However you are collecting data—from interviews, surveys, observations, or document reviews—you will want to organize your information in a logical and accessible format for your readers.

As noted earlier, this is the time to lay out sample blank tables to await your data and analyses. Consider organizing your qualitative data in a spreadsheet or table format for analysis. Quantitative data can be prepared in table format for reviewing descriptive results and then further statistical tests reported. Earlier chapters provide further discussion on analysis plans.

Planning for the Discussion Section

The discussion section serves as a type of commentary. It provides an opportunity to share your interpretation and opinions about your project findings as well as to discuss the implications of your findings. Also you will address these questions: What was accomplished by doing your project? What was gained from learning the specific results? The discussion should also suggest to the reader what action should be taken and what should be done given these findings. Approaches include tying results to the initial review of the literature, relating your findings to the project purpose/questions, identifying implications or the "so what" of your findings, and describing strengths and limitations.

Relating Your Findings to the Project Purpose

Relating your findings back to your purpose statement helps keep your findings focused. You also have the opportunity to relate project findings or outcomes to your initial theories and hypotheses.

Tying Results to the Initial Literature Review

As noted, again plan to consider the literature and describe the similarities or differences found in your project results. This will be the time to put your project findings into the literature-review context.

Identifying Implications of Your Findings

The "so what" approach to findings includes addressing further implications for education, practice, and further research. This includes implications for your populations, patients, staff, and students.

Anticipating the Project Strengths/Limits

Remind yourself to reconsider the strengths/limits of your planned project at this point and document these. Sample description of limits for a small project might include:

> *Limits*: Small descriptive sample results; tested in only one setting
> *Strengths*: Protocol developed from best-evidence literature; expert peer-review panel for protocol review

● ● ●

USING THE ABSTRACT AS A TOOL TO FINALIZE YOUR WORK

The proposal abstract will be the most read and beneficial document of your project, stating clearly in limited space, why the project is important, what is to be done in the study, and potential outcomes and implications. Your abstract will include the key components of your proposal in abbreviated form. It can serve as a checklist that all important components of the Project Triangle (Appendix A) have been addressed. The abstract's abbreviated format also provides an easy communication tool for your team members. Note that a "proposal" abstract is a summary of the proposed project. A "project" abstract is a summary of the completed project. A good abstract will demonstrate significance to practice, methodological soundness, and clear writing.

When you finalize your project, the proposal abstract will be revisited with the opportunity to complete a final project abstract, changing the abstract's verbs to the past tense and filling in the project outcomes and implications. This revision of your initial proposal abstract will address what work has been completed and highlight project results and their implications. Box 15.1 provides an example of a final project abstract. Your abstract should broadly answer the following questions:

- Why did you begin the project?
- What specifically did you do?
- What did you learn?
- What are the implications?

BOX 15.1

FINAL PROJECT ABSTRACT: USING GLUCOSE PATTERNS TO IMPROVE DIABETES MANAGEMENT IN LONG-TERM CARE

Roberta Mansfield, APRN, DNP

The long-term care (LTC) setting often provides systems-level challenges for both facility nurses and primary care providers who manage residents with diabetes. The purpose of this project was to outline the development of a diabetes management module that can be used as a facilitated training resource by staff nurses working in LTC, and to describe the impact of this intervention at the systems level. A 151-bed nursing care facility in the Midwest region of the United States was the site for a quality-improvement project to educate 10 facility nurses on evidence-based practices for interpreting plasma

(continued)

BOX 15.1 *(continued)*

glucose data, identifying trends and patterns, and communicating findings to providers. An instructional module was developed and piloted with nurse managers and staff nurses at the facility. A pre/posttest and module evaluation survey demonstrated positive acquisition of knowledge and skills related to content at the time of implementation. A guided discussion session evaluated the sustainability of this intervention on individual clinical behaviors and the effect at the systems level. Through enhanced awareness and partnership with facility nurses, nurse practitioners will be better able to access and act on information essential to the improvement of glucose control for residents with diabetes.

To convert these questions into a scholarly communication format, the scholarly parts addressed in the abstract should include:

- *Background*: Why was this important? What was your purpose in doing this?
- *Brief literature*: What evidence did you find for the need/approach?
- *Methods*: What did you do? (systematic description) How did you analyze/evaluate?
- *Results*: Placeholder for the outcomes you will gain.
- *Discussion and implications*: Placeholder for discussing why the findings are important to your populations as well as implications for education, practice, and research.

● ● ●

TOOLS THAT FACILITATE PROPOSAL COMPLETION

The Project Team/Committee

Recall that you have developed a team or committee to support you through the clinical project process. Just as the patient is part of his or her own clinical team, you are an important part of your project team/committee. Once you have thoroughly reviewed and edited the proposal, seek your team or committee's review and use their time wisely.

Peer Review

Peer or colleague review of your proposal can be complementary to team and mentor reviews. Seeking input and feedback from others who work with similar situations or topics can be invaluable; this offers another objective review. The review provides an opportunity for further dialogue and more questions. If you serve as a peer reviewer, remember your role includes providing feedback that gives direction as well as offering encouragement and support to your colleague. Benefits of providing peer review include gaining critical-appraisal skills, participating in an interactive process, and practice at providing constructive feedback (Boehm & Bonnel, 2010).

With the opportunity of gaining peer or mentor feedback also comes the responsibility of receiving constructive feedback, reflecting, and responding to that feedback (Leedy & Omrod, 2013). For example, working with mentors in finishing the proposal involves clear communication and responding to feedback on schedule. It also includes being mindful and respectful in use of others' time.

Self-Review and Your Decision Trail

Reflection can provide both a proposal review and a debriefing of proposal/ project experiences. As a proposal review, reflective self-assessment against a standard, such as a proposal rubric, can be a helpful tool for self-accountability. Proposal rubrics, such as those provided in courses or from clinical agencies, serve as a type of guide. This reflective self-assessment can help examine your progress prior to submitting to a mentor for feedback.

Reflection can also serve as a type of debriefing, allowing you to name what you are doing and learning. As you continue your reflective writing and decision trail, remember to write about not only what you are doing, but what barriers you have, how you deal with these, and general thoughts/impressions about how first the proposal, then the project is progressing. Make an effort to extend this experience to a weekly reflection on your work. The ongoing reflective log/decision trail serves as a written reflection to help document project process and analysis. This can be useful as you later write up the final project, serving as a record of thoughts on the implementation process as well as emerging data. Opportunities are gained to focus and facilitate project learning and to promote quality improvement for future projects.

• • •
___

REFLECTING AND SELF-EDITING

Complete a final self-edit as you read your final proposal draft out loud. Are the following concepts evident?

1. Does the challenge/problem grab and convince within the first page?
2. Are precise, consistent words used to describe key concepts?
3. Are unnecessary adjectives deleted such as "extra-special?"
4. Is the third person maintained throughout (or first person if acceptable via guidelines)?
5. Are perfected grammar and spelling in place?
6. Are abbreviations or acronyms used only minimally, if at all?

Your Own Accountability

As you move forward with your clinical project, you will continue to exercise and strengthen skills that have helped you get to this point. Assets, such as accountability and goal setting, will serve you well in finalizing your proposal and moving to the implementation phase of your clinical project. Here are some points to follow to help in being accountable and to further goal setting:

- Avoid the blame game
- Ask relevant questions and use feedback
- Work at problem solving
- Recognize strengths and limitations of a project
- Continue your decision/audit trail

• • •

TURNING THE PROPOSAL INTO A FINISHED PROJECT DOCUMENT

An important goal for the proposal is that it be used as the basis for a completed project. In most cases this involves using the initial sections of the proposal as they stand; the methods section of your proposal is then revised to document completion, meaning verbiage is changed to past tense and any clarifying details of the actual project implementation are added. Results and implications sections, as noted previously, are then completed.

• • •

PRESENTING YOUR PROPOSAL FROM THE PODIUM

In some cases, an oral presentation of the project proposal is required, either to a committee or a broader audience. As with the written proposal, you will want to communicate with others that your project proposal is based on a good idea, uses good evidence, and demonstrates sound approaches (that others might replicate).

You will want to get the attendees' attention, helping them see the importance of the problem and that it needs to be addressed. You will share your proposal, then at a later date, your finished project story. This will include thoughts on why you did this, what you did, what happened/outcomes, and "now what" components.

Your verbal proposal, often guided by a PowerPoint presentation will address the who, what, where, and when of your proposal plans. Even if individuals have read a proposal copy, the verbal presentation provides an opportunity to remind and focus participants on the key components. A sample format for proposal slides for a PowerPoint presentation is provided in Appendix 15.1.

Also learn from the experience of doctor of nursing practice (DNP) students who have completed proposals. Their advice is presented in the following box.

• • •

ADVICE FROM DNP STUDENTS

Finalizing Project Writing

Create your proposal in parts and seek feedback on each part
- Receiving feedback on the parts (or sections) is very helpful prior to completing the full task.

Be prepared for multiple revisions
- Numerous revisions are normal, even for people who have been doing this a while.

Allow time for edits and rewriting
- The proposal process contains many revisions.
- The rewriting is very time consuming, I kept thinking, "Gosh, I hope I am getting closer to a proposal."
- I learned why it was necessary to reevaluate and rewrite, and rewrite and rewrite.

Keep referring back to the project triangle
- The most important thing that I learned while completing my proposal was always to refer back to my project triangle to stay focused.

There is no such thing as a perfect paper
- Put ideas on paper as best you can; then consult your mentor.

SUMMARY

The proposal serves as a valuable communication tool, necessitating clear written communication that is central to scholarly work. Completing the proposal involves gaining better writing skills, not only planning project methods, but clearly conveying them. The value of gaining new tools for writing/completing the clinical project proposal and reflecting on what has been accomplished is a part of this. Considering next steps in implementing the proposal helps move toward project completion and contributes to quality patient care outcomes.

NEXT CHAPTER UP

How do you move forward with your proposal-implementation plans? What next steps exist for using your proposal? The next chapter helps you address these questions.

LEARNING ACTIVITIES

To-Do List

A final proposal check:

1. Is the full document packaged professionally as a scholarly document? Does it follow a systematic approach? Appropriate metrics? Reasonable analysis plans? Do you have plans for tables and graphs to clearly convey future findings?
2. Has your proposal been peer reviewed (by colleagues, mentor, project team)?
3. Have you written summaries of each proposal section for clarity? Is the finished proposal written in scholarly format?

_____

_____

_____

_____

_____

_____

_____

_____

REFERENCES

Boehm, H., & Bonnel, W. (2010). The use of peer review in nursing education and clinical practice. *Journal of Nursing Staff Development, 26*(3), 108–115.

Bonnel, D. (2011). *Physical therapist assistant students' attitudes towards electronic health records* (Unpublished senior project). Washburn University, Topeka, KS.

Galvan, J. (2013). *Writing literature reviews: A guide for students of the social and behavioural sciences* (5th ed.). London, UK: Routledge.

Leedy, P., & Omrod, J. (2013). *Practical research: Planning and design* (10th ed.). Boston, MA: Pearson.

APPENDIX 15.1

SAMPLE FORMAT FOR A POWERPOINT PRESENTATION OF THE PROPOSAL

The following sample slides for a "created" study follow a basic abstract format and might serve as a template or at least ideas for a PowerPoint presentation of your proposal.

Slide 1: Title: New Graduate Perceptions of Readiness to Use Electronic Health Records
Author: W. Brown

Slide 2: Thanks to committee members . . .

Slide 3: My background . . . As a DNP student on a clinical leadership track, I really enjoy working with new graduates in my clinical specialty area and hope to guide them in projects such as use of electronic health records (EHRs).

Slide 4: What brought me to this project . . . I was concerned by the number of challenges I was seeing when new graduates reached the clinical setting related to EHRs. EHRs are relatively new, but they are key to patient safety and interdisciplinary communication.

Slide 5: What was the purpose . . . The purpose of this project was to survey graduating students on their perceptions and perceived readiness to use EHRs.

Slide 6: Brief literature review . . .
I found some medical literature about beginning graduate use of EHRs but very limited studies were available in nursing or other disciplines. The most valuable studies were . . .

Slide 7: Methods
- This will be a descriptive survey administered at one setting.
- Graduating seniors will be surveyed at a final class session.
- Consent for the study will be attained by the school's Human Subjects Committee.

Slide 8: The Survey
- The surveys to be used are adapted from the Bonnel (2011) EHR Survey and Brief Demographic Data Tool.
- The Bonnel EHR survey was adapted from two descriptive surveys in the literature.

- The EHR survey has two open-ended questions and 12 closed-ended items for participant rating, with a 1-4 (high) scale.
- A sample item is "I am adequately proficient in EHR skills."
- The survey will be piloted with three junior students to support clarity.

Slide 9: Methods (*continued*)
- A letter of invitation to the graduates along with the surveys will be provided to all graduating seniors at the close of one class.
- All surveys will be collected in a large box by a second faculty member.

Slide 10: Analysis
- Descriptive statistics for *demographic* data will be completed and a table of descriptive sample characteristics created.
- Descriptive statistics for survey *closed-ended items* will be completed and a summary table created.
- Common themes from content analysis will be identified from *open-ended responses* and exemplars provided.

Slide 11: Project Strengths/Limitations
- Strengths include the benefits of gaining graduates' perceptions via survey data.
- Limitations include the fact there is just one sample and one setting and they may not represent the full graduate population.

Slide 12: Potential Project Implications
For Practice: Gaining new graduates' perceptions of EHR knowledge may lead to ideas for orienting new graduates in EHR use.
- For Education: Further education may be recommended in the student setting.
- For Further Research: Further study of the best ways to learn and use EHRs may be indicated.

Slide 13: Thanks to committee; thanks to audience members for their interest.

Slide 14: Questions?

16

· · ·

Keeping Your Advanced Clinical Project Proposal Going

Reflective Questions

In Chapter 15, you focused on gaining better writing skills to complete your written proposal, focusing on how to clearly convey your project plans. In this final chapter, you will focus on the "what next" for your completed proposal. The following reflective questions guide this chapter. With which of the following are you most comfortable?

- Reflecting on what's been gained?
- Considering next steps in implementing and evaluating the proposal?
- Considering next steps in completing and sharing the completed proposal project?

This chapter is about pulling the entire project together. It allows you the opportunity to stop and celebrate the accomplishment of a well-written proposal. It encourages reflecting on the big picture of what has been learned in developing this proposal and reflecting on what still needs to be done.

The advanced clinical project has helped you name and focus your area of expertise. This chapter comes full circle to create proposals for projects that enhance safe, quality patient care for diverse populations and settings. Using best practices to gain mentoring, peer review, and self-assessment will help continue to achieve these objectives. Additional focus includes reflective opportunities for expanding clinical scholarship and interprofessional team opportunities. Implementing the proposal and completing the project then lead to opportunities for sharing/disseminating your work and developing further projects. The proposal will be used as a component of a final paper reporting on your complete project.

• • •

THE PROPOSAL: REFLECTING ON WHAT HAS BEEN GAINED

Clinical Scholarship Models

The clinical project proposal provides an opportunity to extend scholarship to the clinical setting. The Boyer (1990) model focuses on scholarship in four broad domains; clinical projects often relate to the scholarship of application. Boyer describes the scholarship of application as applying knowledge from theory, practice, and research to address goals related to client outcomes, community concerns, and environmental challenges.

The American Association of Colleges of Nursing (AACN; 2006), in its doctorate of nursing practice (DNP) essentials, discusses forms of scholarship as including the clinical project. Through gaining proposal skills, you have gained skills such as those described in the DNP graduate competencies, including methods to:

- Review and synthesize the best evidence for practice
- Develop projects to evaluate practice at varied levels from patient to populations and systems
- Use quality-improvement tools to enhance practice
- Use best evidence to guide protocol development to enhance patient care
- Use technology to gain data to better understand patient care process and outcomes and generate further projects

Clinical Scholarship and National Agendas

Expanding clinical scholarship provides the opportunity to enhance the profession. National organizations, such as the Quality and Safety Education for Nurses program (Cronenwett et al., 2009) and the Institute of Medicine's (2003), Health Professions Education Report provide broad direction as to important themes needed to achieve safe, quality care. Projects that address themes such as these contribute to clinical scholarship and the nursing profession's knowledge base. The following summarize themes within these resources.

- *Evidence-based practice*: The focus on evidence has been emphasized throughout this text. Reflect on how your proposal will help extend the use of evidence in practice. Consistent with guides for DNP scholarship (AACN, 2006), this is central to the work of all advanced practice nurses.
- *Technology*: Rapid advances in electronic health records and various clinical databases provide new opportunities for gaining data to better understand patient populations and their needs as well as to document outcomes. Opportunities to gain data via provider, patient, and technology interfaces offer opportunities to advance scholarship. Using technology to its fullest potential can include creative use of newer technologies that facilitate both staff and patient interventions and data collection.
- *Collaborative work*: Optimizing the use of interprofessional teams is a central component of the agenda to improve health care. Teamwork included in team-supported clinical projects is an essential component of patient-centered care. Recently, interprofessional competencies that include clear communication and scholarship have been developed to help move this effort forward (Interprofessional Education Collaborative, 2011).
- *Quality improvement*: The essence of advanced clinical projects is improving quality care. Clinical projects have the potential to lead to changes in systems and to enhance quality and safety. In today's data-driven world, scholarly skills gained in proposal writing and project completion are key components for future lifelong learning and evidence-based practice.
- *Patient-centered care*: Opportunities to gain the patients' perspective of what quality care means to them. Focus on safety is a key component of relevant clinical projects as well.

* * *

NEXT STEPS: USING THE PROPOSAL

Although this book is about proposal writing, providing a "hint" to the next project phases is appropriate. Once the hard work of pulling together multiple pieces of your proposal is accomplished and approved, then the next steps begin. Next steps involve project implementation/evaluation, writing the final report, and continuing scholarly plans for project dissemination.

Implementing/Evaluating

A successful proposal gets you to the exciting part of your project: its actual implementation and evaluation. As you think forward to the next steps of your project, major components include adhering to project protocols, continuing team communication, and working professionally with all team members.

Adhering to Project Protocols as You Implement and Evaluate Your Proposal

At this point, you have laid out your plans; hence, all involved know what is going on. Now it is your responsibility to stay true to your plans. In large part, thus far this has included clear documentation of approved project plans/ processes. If unforeseen challenges should occur, you need to communicate with your team about any needed protocol changes and to confirm any alternate plans. Any changes will include communication with your institutional review board as well.

Another way to document that you are staying true to your plans is achieved in part by keeping decision or audit trails. These tools also serve as timelines and journals of not only what is being done, but also why choices are being made.

Continuing Communication and Working Professionally With Team Members

Your proposal is a contract with your project committee or other team members. It provides the detail for keeping others on track (clarifying who will do what and when). Proposal implementation also involves meeting professional standards in working with the team, including clear communication and monitoring team function. Clinical project teamwork may include direct involvement with patients, working with staff to enhance protocols/approaches, or working with larger unit/system approaches to enhance safe/quality patient care. As a clinical leader, you will have opportunities to guide staff in evidence-based projects. You will want a proposal that is clear and concise to share with the team; one that conveys your plan to help document clinical outcomes and to improve structure and process as needed.

• • •

NEXT STEPS: FINAL REPORT WRITE-UP

Your proposal will become part of the early sections of your final paper, in which you report on your completed project. The final sections in scholarly documents are the results and then the discussion/implications section. As noted previously, the results section of a paper contains "just the facts." It is a detailing of the data that was gained in an organized meaningful presentation of what was learned. The final section of the traditional scholarly paper includes the discussion/implications information. In this section, the findings are considered from the "so what" perspective. In other words, what do these findings mean? Your well-written proposal can lead to a strong finished project with potential benefits to safe, quality patient care.

NEXT STEPS: ADVANCING WITH CONTINUED CLINICAL SCHOLARSHIP

The importance of supporting lifelong learning for all health professionals has been acknowledged (Institute of Medicine, 2011). This includes ongoing learning by proposing and completing clinical projects; such scholarly projects can become a key part of learning. Recall that the project proposal is also a tool used to prepare for future work in advanced clinical leadership. Clinical project proposal writing serves as a bridge to advanced clinical leadership. Project proposals can lead to:

- Future presentations/publications
- Proposals for future grant writing
- Opportunities for further clinical projects

The Value of the Reflective Portfolio in Further Project Write-Up

A reflective portfolio that documents your proposal journey can be a major tool in furthering your project scholarship. Portfolios provide opportunity for packaging activities and naming what you do in your clinical scholarship. The portfolio is a tool to promote reflection and communication about accomplishments. A portfolio that documents each of the sections of your proposal can showcase your ongoing clinical project progress and document one component of your clinical expertise. The benefits of portfolios include helping document/ track components with other team members and sharing with others the scholarship that is developed in a clinical setting. They also serve as a way to document clinical scholarship via naming and describing knowledge gained and supporting generation of questions that require further study.

Adding a reflective component to your portfolio, or a summary of your perspectives as to accomplishments and lessons learned, serves as a way to share your specific story about purposes and strategies for projects that advance safe, quality patient care. Your final, reflective summary provides opportunity to reinforce your key points and the benefit of a successful project. A reflective portfolio helps you think about the big-picture process of your proposal (as you progress and as you finish) and helps prepare for future work in clinical proposal writing. It reminds you to consider what was gained using the approaches selected and how that may be valuable in future clinical projects. It also reminds you to address what surprised you, or what you would you do differently in a future project, essentially preparing you for the "what next?" A portfolio of your proposal, and later your project, helps support:

- Reflection on what you do
- Communication with others about what you do
- Ownership of the work and learning that has been accomplished
- Value in helping document this lengthy project
- Organization for further project scholarship

Completing the Project and Planning for Publication

Scholarship models include dissemination of scholarly work. According to Huber and Hutchings (2005), projects must be peer reviewed and passed on via public venues such as publications. Oermann and Hays (2011) summarize reasons to publish that include sharing expertise, disseminating new evidence, gaining advancement (in both education and clinical settings), developing your own knowledge and skills, and achieving your own satisfaction. Those in diverse advanced clinician roles in particular have reason, even obligation, to write and share knowledge gained related to improving patient care. Just as in proposal writing, revising a final project, to suit publication format, will include creating a timeline. This timeline will include selecting the appropriate journal, outlining the manuscript, and writing according to the journal's guidelines.

Proposals for Future Grant Writing

As advanced clinicians there will be future opportunities to write proposals and gain resources to document scholarship with populations of interest. In learning proposal-writing skills, you have also gained tools for critiquing and synthesizing the literature, created worksheets for laying out the big-picture plans, and created templates for mapping out future projects. Concepts used in proposal writing and in creating sections of proposals apply across all scholarly venues. You have gained a toolkit of resources to help document and make the case for future projects. The potential for grant funding exists with well-written proposals.

Proposals for Further Clinical Projects

The initial project proposal often serves as a tool for reflecting and learning as the basis for generating further projects. In considering future plans, recall that project proposals help communicate about what you do as an advanced clinician and address further goal setting or "what's next?" with your specialty. The project may lead to using project methods in further venues and to extending expertise with your specialty population. Advanced clinicians have opportunities to practice with unique populations. These projects can help others better understand these populations and serve as tools for mentoring others.

* * *

ADDITIONAL CONCEPTS OF VALUE

Developing and Continuing the Mentor Partnership

Throughout the development of your proposal, you will be working with a mentor of some type. It is likely you will gain informal mentoring from individuals related to your project, as well as from a more formal mentor. The best use of resources is to find a mentor whose interests already match yours or are closely related. This provides a type of incentive for all to eagerly move forward. Your mentoring relationship will benefit from clear communication, both written and verbal. It should also involve fair, equitable use of both mentor and mentee time.

Reflection serves as a key concept of mentoring. Reflection allows you to make explicit to your mentor what you are doing and learning. Your portfolio serves as a product to help you move forward in your career. Reflecting on first your proposal and then your project accomplishments may help lead to success in future projects This reflection can help analyze experiences with the goal of improving work, but also at proposal completion there is value in reflecting and celebrating this milestone achieved.

In many cases, you will stay connected with faculty mentors after the proposal is completed. You may consider renegotiating for future work. Mentor and mentee roles may even coexist as you share your unique clinical expertise with your mentor in future projects. Additional possibilities include moving on to another mentor or considering whether you are ready to take on the mentoring role yourself.

Caring for Self and Having a Peer Group

Staying motivated to complete a big project involves caring for oneself. Remember to create time and space to care for yourself as well as focusing on your scholarship. This includes creating time and activities for physical and emotional health as well. Colleagues or peer groups can play a role in this process as well. Peers can help in debriefing project activities and help you stay motivated to complete your project. Peer groups can be formalized to include scheduled journal club–type activities or be maintained in informal venues.

● ● ●
_____

CONTINUING SELF-ASSESSMENT AND REFLECTION

Scholarship and mindful clinical practice go hand in hand. You have reflected as you completed the proposal; learning through reflection and reflecting on learning will enhance future work. Using reflective journaling has been a key concept in your proposal writing. At each stage of proposal writing, as you have made choices that further directed your work, you have addressed the basic questions of what, so what, now what? Now, as you finish your proposal, reflecting on the full process and product provides opportunities to cement learning and gain a basis for future ideas and plans. Here are some reflective prompts to guide thoughts on your proposal work:

1. Why was this work important to you?
2. What was the most important thing that you learned from creating this proposal?
3. How does this proposal help you document what you do as an advanced clinician?
4. What was it like for you to create this proposal? What most surprised you about your work on this proposal?
5. What did you gain from creating this proposal? What new skills or strategies were acquired?

6. How did this proposal work expand your previous knowledge? How did this advance your thinking about the topic or subject area?
7. How did this work enhance your role as an advanced clinician?
8. How will you be able to use what you gained from this experience in future work as an advanced clinician?
9. If you were to continue your work on this product, what further approaches would you consider?
10. What further learning goals do you have related to this work?

SUMMARY

Proposal-writing skills are important for nurses to develop. You have created a proposal for a project of interest. Whether administrative, clinical, staff developmental, or other, your proposal has been guided by the best evidence available as you considered the theories and models available. Your blend of knowledge, motivation, and the setting of your research will likely lead to further work as you implement, finalize, and then share your project with others.

Being an expert clinician comes with the responsibility of scholarship. Once the proposal is implemented, the opportunity exists to further package and disseminate your learning. Gaining tools for scholarly writing provides the beginning of your journey. Creating a portfolio showcasing the entire project helps package and lay the groundwork for further presentation/publication. Good proposals can lead to good projects. Results of these important clinical projects then lead to developing practice improvements and helping to direct the future of patient care.

REFERENCES

American Association of Colleges of Nursing. (2006). The essentials of doctoral education for advanced nursing practice. Retrieved from http://www.aacn.nche.edu/dnp/pdf/essentials.pdf

Boyer, E. L. (1990). *Scholarship reconsidered: Priorities of the professoriate.* Princeton, NJ: Carnegie Foundation for the Advancement of Teaching.

Cronenwett, L., Sherwood, G., Pohl, J., Barnsteiner, J., Moore, S., Sullivan, D. T., . . . Warren, J. (2009). Quality and safety education for advanced nursing practice. *Nursing Outlook, 57*(6), 338–348.

Huber, M., & Hutchings, P. (2005). *The advancement of learning: Building the teaching commons.* San Francisco, CA: Jossey-Bass.

Institute of Medicine. (2011). *The future of nursing: Leading change, advancing health.* Washington, DC: National Academies Press.

Institute of Medicine Committee on the Health Professions Education. (2003). *Health professions education: A bridge to quality.* Washington, DC: National Academies Press.

Interprofessional Education Collaborative. (2011). Core competencies for interprofessional collaborative practice. Retrieved from http://www.aacn.nche.edu/education-resources/ipecreport.pdf

Oermann, M., & Hays, H. (2011). *Writing for publication in nursing* (2nd ed.). New York, NY: Springer Publishing.

Appendices

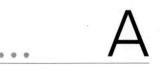

Project Triangle Model

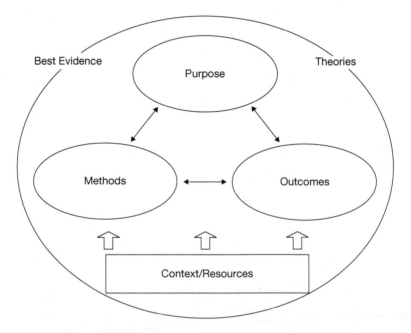

Once you have clearly identified the project problem, you are ready to use components of this model to develop your proposal. The checklist in Appendix B assists you in reflecting on your work.

B

Checklist for Planning or Self-Assessment of a Specific Project

As you move forward with your project proposal, check to see whether you have adequately addressed each of the following. Note "agree" or "disagree" to confirm that each area has been thoroughly considered.

Concept	Have You Considered	Agree/ Disagree
Evidence-based practice	What evidence is available to guide initiating and implementing a particular project?	
Theory or conceptual model	What theories might best fit in guiding the project?	
Logistics/context with assessment of unit/setting	Have you assessed the need for your project?	
	Have you assessed feasibility of your project?	
	What are the facilitators/barriers for completing the project in a specific setting?	
Purpose	Does the purpose flow from the identified problem?	
	What is to be achieved with the project?	
Methods	Have you reviewed diverse potential approaches to your problem?	
	What is the best approach for your given problem and project purpose?	

(continued)

(continued)

Concept	Have You Considered	Agree/ Disagree
Outcomes evaluation	What are your project outcomes to be evaluated?	
	How will you know your project is successful?	
Reflective review/ critique	What are the strengths and weaknesses of your proposal?	
	Are there points you can strengthen?	

C

Proposal Abstract: Improving the Care of Patients With Chronic Kidney Disease Using Evidence-Based Guidelines

Gwenyth Wagner

PROBLEM STATEMENT

There is a documented gap between best evidence guidelines and implementation of these guidelines in the care of chronic kidney disease (CKD) patients in primary care.

PURPOSE

To develop and implement a quality-improvement survey that can be used to evaluate adherence to clinical guidelines for the care of patients with CKD and ultimately suggest approaches to improve translation of evidence-based care into practice.

* * *

CONTEXT

The setting will be a Midwest primary care clinic.

* * *

METHODS

- A quality-improvement tool will be developed to measure practice-level clinical performance data.
- Clinical performance measures will be derived from the Kidney Disease Quality Outcomes Initiative (KDQOI) guidelines.
- A chart review of approximately 50 patients with a glomerular filtration rate (GFR) less than 60 will be conducted using the clinical performance tool.
- A talking-points summary will be developed to share best practice guidelines, results of the chart review, and an evaluation of the quality-improvement tool with the medical director and other staff as appropriate.

D

Proposal Abstract: Improving Diabetes Care Delivery in an Integrated Health Clinic

Jane Robinson

People with serious mental illness (SMI), as a population, are typically underserved and likely to have barriers to accessing primary care services. When these patients do seek primary care, it is often fragmented and communication between multiple providers lacks efficiency and coordination. A colocated primary care clinic was recently established in a large behavioral health setting to improve access to primary care for this population. Prior to opening the clinic, in a survey of 499 client respondents, 82 indicated they needed help managing their diabetes. Multiple providers with varied backgrounds are providing care in the new clinic setting where potential gaps in the delivery of diabetes-related care are likely. The purpose of this project is to evaluate the care provided to patients with type 2 diabetes mellitus in the primary care clinic by multiple providers compared to a standard. The standard will be medical care for diabetes management according to the American Diabetes Association (ADA) 2015 guidelines. A retrospective chart review using a standards checklist based on the ADA guidelines will be used to evaluate care provided by a number of different providers. The intent is to identify any gaps in care. Feedback will be shared with providers in a post study discussion. Implications may include the potential for improvements in documentation and use of the checklist as a tool to improve delivery of care.

E

Project Abstract: Unit-Based Council Chairs' Perception of Unit-Based Councils

Sonya Curtis

BACKGROUND

Nurse managers are consistently dealing with day-to-day operational management of the microsystem for which they are held accountable and responsible. Nurse managers are not always visible on the unit, at the point of care, to know what the patients need for maintaining the plan of care that has been set forth. Staff nurses are verbalizing frustrations with their lack of autonomy regarding decision making at the bedside and changing current professional clinical practice. This critical problem is impacting nurse job satisfaction, intent to leave, and patient care. Literature suggests that nurse managers should make every effort to ensure that nurses are exposed to high-quality work environments, which in turn increase their organizations' ability to attract and retain nurses. Leaders are urged to collaborate with staff nurses to create work environments that maximize their ability to provide optimal care to patients. The literature suggests introducing an element of shared governance, which is a unit-based council (UBC).

246

● ● ●

PURPOSE

The purpose of this quality-improvement project was to evaluate UBC chairs' perception of UBCs.

● ● ●

METHOD

This quality as noted improvement project surveyed a sample of 37 RNs, who are UBC chairs, from a large Midwest academic medical center. The UBC Perceptions Survey, consisting of five open-ended questions, assessed broadly the UBC chairs' perception of the functioning of their UBC. The UBCs Functionality Measurement Tool was utilized to evaluate more directly the perception of UBCs' functioning. This tool has 21 items indicating characteristics of a successful UBC.

● ● ●

FINDINGS AND CONCLUSIONS

A majority of respondents (N = 29/37) reported the UBCs to be high functioning. Qualitative themes supported participants' appreciation of the UBC with themes, including valuing the UBC, improving patient outcomes, feeling appreciated, improving nursing practice, and having a voice. Aggregate data from surveys will be used to provide feedback to the UBC chairs with the goal of quality improvement related to UBCs. Project findings support the value of UBCs in hospital practice and decision making for nurses participating in UBCs at the point of care.

F

Proposal Abstract: Evidence Generating: Learning From Practitioner Owners of Clinics in Missouri

Paula Israel

BACKGROUND

In Missouri, a collaborative practice agreement is required for nurse practitioners (NPs) to deliver care. Delegated tasks are more restrictive than what is possible based on education and scope of practice granted by the state board of nursing. In addition, limitations are imposed by legislators in Missouri.

SIGNIFICANCE

A dearth of providers has created unprecedented opportunities for NPs. Existing literature cites limited autonomy, reduced rates of reimbursement, incongruent state practice acts, and lack of business acumen as barriers to independent NP clinic ownership. NPs are identified as one viable solution to the lack of primary care providers in the United States.

• • •

PURPOSE

Opportunities and barriers to NP-owned clinics will be explored through the review of the literature and by description of experiences of NP clinic owners in one Midwestern state.

• • •

THEORY

Donabedian's theory of structure, process, and outcomes provides a framework for this project. Regulations and reimbursement (structure) allowing NPs to practice to the full extent of their training (process) could increase health care access (outcome) for Missourians.

• • •

METHODS

This will be a descriptive, exploratory study of NP clinic owners. An online survey, consisting of 11 open-ended and four structured questions, was developed from the literature and insights were gained from observing one business owner's patterns and practices. Fourteen of 19 identified clinic owners will meet inclusion criteria and be invited to describe their experience through self-report.

• • •

ANALYSIS

Descriptive analysis will include a summary of participant characteristics. Content analysis of qualitative data responses will be completed seeking key themes. Implications for practice, policy, education, and research will be generated from the findings.

G

Proposal Abstract: Evidence Synthesis: Anesthesia Considerations and Implications for Obese Pediatric Patients

Karri Arndt

The number of Americans described as being overweight or obese has been increasing at an alarming rate over the past 30 years. Overweight and obesity in both children and adults have been identified not only by the United States Department of Health and Human Services, Centers for Disease Control (2009) as an epidemic in the United States, but also as a pandemic by the World Health Organization (WHO; 2009). The WHO (2009) states that childhood obesity is one of the most serious public health challenges of the 21st century. As the rate of overweight and obese individuals increases, so does the economic burden of obesity-related health care in the United States and worldwide.

Many diseases that were once thought to be present only in adults are now being seen in children and teenagers. These include cardiovascular disease, hypertension, elevated cholesterol levels, diabetes, insulin resistance, metabolic syndrome, musculoskeletal disorders, osteoarthritis, certain types of cancers, and sleep apnea. Concerns specific to anesthesia include obstructive sleep apnea, difficult mask ventilation, difficult intubation, and asthma. These comorbid conditions are known to increase the risk associated with anesthesia and are a growing concern among pediatric anesthesia providers.

Ambulatory surgery centers are also seeing a greater number of obese pediatric patients in their facilities for what are typically considered minor to moderate outpatient procedures. However, the presence of these comorbid conditions is making safe care a challenge in these facilities as anesthesia providers do not have the same ancillary resources, invasive equipment, difficult-airway devices, or various medical services readily available in the event of a complication or emergency. These facilities also are not equipped for overnight stays should perioperative complications arise. It is imperative that anesthesia providers have a thorough understanding of the anesthetic implications and unique challenges associated with the obese pediatric population.

The purpose of this project is to review the current literature related to perioperative morbidity, mortality, issues, and concerns that arise when caring for obese pediatric patients requiring anesthesia services to prepare an educational resource and an article for submission to the American Association of Nurse Anesthetists (AANA) professional journal.

A comprehensive review article using the most current evidence-based data will describe the prevalence of obesity in children, identify coexisting diseases and their management, discuss pharmacokinetic and pharmacodynamic considerations, identify anesthetic management techniques for this unique patient population, and identify specific questions that require further research. The purpose of the article is to increase awareness of pediatric obesity and its implications and improve knowledge and competency of anesthesia providers, which will better prepare them to safely handle increasing numbers of obese children, especially in the ambulatory setting. More specific research is needed in this area, and an article of this nature is intended to stimulate thought, provoke questions, and motivate providers to initiate such research and disseminate their findings to improve perioperative management of this complex patient population.

● ● ●

METHODOLOGY

The methodology for collecting data and information for this project will include an exhaustive review of the literature located in PubMed, Cumulative Index to Nursing and Allied Health Literature (CINAHL) using the key terms: "pediatric, obesity, anesthesia, morbidity, and mortality." Other sources to be searched include the American Society of Anesthesiologists, the AANA, the Society for Pediatric Anesthesia, and current anesthesia text and reference books, using the same key-word searches. The Centers for Disease Control will be searched for current statistical data related to the prevalence of and trends in childhood obesity.

Information obtained from the database searches will be reviewed and critically assessed for relevance and reliability. References in high-quality studies will also be reviewed for potential relevant material. Obtained data will then be organized in an easy-to-review database matrix that will identify the reference citation, type of article or research conducted, evidence obtained, key points, and limitations. Information will then be combined into a concise educational resource and review article for submission. These resources will provide a literature synthesis with discussion of state-of-the-art information, summary of the anesthetic implications associated with the perioperative care of obese pediatric patients, and recommendations for future research.

H

Proposal Abstract: Evidence Implementing and Testing: Improving the Communication of Clinical Information Between Nurses and Physicians in Long-Term Care

Linda Kroeger

Based on personal observation; experience in receiving calls from long-term care (LTC) facilities; and conversations with physicians, registered nurses (RNs), and licensed practical nurses (LPNs) who expressed frustration with their phone interactions, a brief needs assessment was done regarding nurse/ provider calls to and from LTC facilities. Several LPNs reported that their biggest fear was calling to speak with a physician regarding a change in a patient's condition because they lacked confidence in their ability to answer questions asked by the physician.

• • •

PURPOSE

The purpose of this quality-improvement (QI) project is to use developed methods, established protocols, and structured communication techniques to develop and implement a program to teach LTC nurses, including RNs and

LPNs, how to efficiently and competently collect and communicate clinical information to physicians.

* * *

SETTING

A request for participation in this QI project will be made to the director of nursing of a local nursing home. The nursing home consists of six units; each unit has 16 beds and the facility capacity is 96 residents. The facility provides long-term residential care and skilled-nursing care.

* * *

SAMPLE

The nursing staff at this LTC facility is composed of RNs and LPNs. RNs include the director of nursing, the assistant director of nursing, and two Minimum Data Set nurses.

An RN and two LPNs staff the LTC unit on the day and evening shifts, and two LPNs are responsible for the night shift. The nursing home also has nurses who work on call and other LPNs available. The number of RNs and LPNs who will be invited to participate in this QI program for communication training is approximately 13.

* * *

QI PLAN

The training program for communication techniques will begin with an introduction on organizational tips to consider before calling the physician. This will be followed by instruction on the use of the situation, background, assessment, recommendation (SBAR) communication technique. The SBAR method has the support of the Institute for Healthcare Improvement and The Joint Commission. SBAR is an established, evidence-based method shown to be effective in improving clinical communication skills (American Medical Directors Association [AMDA], 2009; Dunsford, 2009). This part of the training program will be made into a PowerPoint presentation with voiceover that could be used for future staff development training programs. Protocol cards, developed by AMDA for use by LTC nurses, are designed to facilitate the gathering and presentation of information during physician phone calls. The 15 most common clinical problems, for example pain and agitation, and their protocol cards will be included in a handout. The AMDA protocol cards will be reviewed, and an example using one card to evaluate a clinical problem, will be demonstrated. A survey measuring nurse satisfaction with telephone communication (10 items) will be administered to LTC nurses before the program, immediately postprogram, and 4 to 6 weeks after instruction. A Wilcoxon signed-rank test will be used to assess for differences.

Index